Children Need Groups

AUP titles of related interest

ROLE PLAY a practical guide
Ellice Milroy

GROWING UP AND GOING OUT
Leo Hendry

OUT TO PLAY
the middle years of childhood
Alasdair Roberts

TELL THEM FROM ME
*edited and introduced by Lesley Gow
and Andrew McPherson*

THE BEST YEARS?
reflections of school leavers in the 1980s
editor Joan Hughes

FOURTEEN TO EIGHTEEN
the changing pattern of schooling in Scotland
editor David Raffe

Children Need Groups

a practical manual for group work with young children

W R SILVEIRA
GILL TRAFFORD

Groups for the sexually abused child
by Rosemarie Musgrave

ABERDEEN UNIVERSITY PRESS

First published 1988
Aberdeen University Press
A member of the Pergamon Group

© W R Silveira, Gill Trafford, Rosemarie Musgrave 1988

All Rights Reserved. No part of this publication may be reproduced, stored in a retrieval system or transmitted in any form or by any means: electronic, electrostatic, magnetic tape, mechanical, photocopying, recording or otherwise, without permission in writing from the copyright holders.

British Library Cataloguing in Publication Data

Silveira, W Raza
    Children need groups : a practical manual for group work with young children.
    1. Children. Group therapy.
    I. Title   II. Trafford, Gill;
    618.92′89152.

    ISBN 0 08 036413 6 (hard)
    ISBN 0 08 036414 4 (flexi)

PRINTED IN GREAT BRITAIN
THE UNIVERSITY PRESS
ABERDEEN

This book is dedicated to
Sue and Richard

Foreword

The title of this book is also its thesis—namely, belonging to an organised peer-group of play-mates can enhance the social and emotional development of young children, provided the group-leaders know what they are about. This special kind of 'knowing' is compounded of natural aptitude and learning by experience, yet surprisingly little has been published about this kind of group-work, which makes this publication particularly timely. The approach, though it could have been written only by those with much clinical experience, is essentially practical and straightforward, and aims at those who work with largely unselected groups of young children in the community and elsewhere. Each chapter has a theme with practical examples of play-strategies for use by group-leaders, with some amusing illustrations. I commend this original and useful text particularly to those who work with pre-school play-groups, mother and toddler groups, infant and primary schoolteachers, residential child-care staff, and hospital play-leaders.

Frederick H Stone
Emeritus Professor of Child &
Adolescent Psychiatry
University of Glasgow

Contents

Foreword by Frederick H Stone		iii
Acknowledgements		xi
1	Introduction	1
2	Parents and toddlers need groups too!	6
3	Stepping into the world of the nursery school	15
4	How do I look?	24
5	Society invites you to join its ranks	38
6	The trauma of *loss*	53
7	Hospitals can be quite nice places really	65
8	Coping with handicap	80
9	Groups on the school timetable	90
10	We live in groups—*residential schools*	100
11	On being a member of the community	111
12	Groups for the sexually abused child	117
Appendices		130
Further Reading		134

Acknowledgements

We would like to thank our colleagues at the Department of Child and Family Psychiatry, R.H.S.C., Glasgow, who took the time to read and comment on the draft manuscript and who made valuable suggestions on form and content.

We are grateful to Mrs Rosemarie Musgrave, Senior Careworker at the Coventry Child Guidance Centre for her contribution to this book, in describing her work with young sexually abused children.

We are especially grateful to Professor Fred Stone for writing the Foreword and for his very helpful comments on the book.

Thanks also to Peter Sandover for his illustrations, and to Mary Crouch (Occupational Therapist).

Our special thanks to Jeanette Tweedlie and Halina Johnson for typing the manuscript.

Raza Silveira
Gill Trafford

1 Introduction

That 'children need groups' is neither a new nor a revolutionary concept. After all, children spend most of their time in groups, be this with the family, in the community or at school. It follows, therefore, that it is important for the child to maintain an acceptable group membership and this is both a learned as well as an instinctive process. The instinctive process is part of man's heritage, his need to live in groups in order to survive. The learning process starts early, in the bosom of the family and in the reciprocity of family life. Learning continues in the socialisation of the child in the parent and toddler group, at nursery school and finally at school itself. A process of shaping occurs that guides the natural tendency of the infant to play alone at first, then in parallel and later to engage in co-operative play when the rules become complex and a system evolves of give and take. The progress through childhood into adolescence and later adult life is again marked by subtle shifts of emphasis in terms of the norms and expectations that the group and the individual hold of each other. A satisfactory conclusion to the learning process is the ultimate ability of the individual to retain his own sense of identity while, at the same time, being able to share in the common interests of the many groups that he finally comes to belong to.

The child who finds it difficult to relate within groups can usually have this difficulty traced back to traumatic events occurring at crucial stages in the development of group social skills. Thus, life events, such as moving home, changing schools, physical illness, separation or loss in the family, etc, etc, occurring at times when the child is just about to negotiate the next rung on the ladder of the group hierarchy, can hinder the child's progress or cause him to regress to earlier and, therefore, inappropriate age behaviours. The child may suffer further from having problems not only in one group, for instance, but across the whole spectrum of other groups that he belongs to.

Group work is one of several approaches to assessment and treatment of children in difficulty. It can be used as an adjunct to individual therapy, with family therapy or be used as a therapeutic medium in its own right. As a form of assessment, group work offers a structure and format in which observations can be made of a child's interaction with his peers, his relationship with adults, his personal likes, dislikes and preoccupations, his characteristic ways of responding to given situations, his views of himself and others, his physical and social abilities, and all the other facets of personality and interaction that do not become readily obvious in the setting of individual and family assessments.

Group work as a treatment mode offers the kind of setting in which situations with which the child is coping badly can be symbolically replicated by a process of directive and structured group exercises and games, socio-drama and art work. Enactment of conflictual situations such as the bully/victim scenario, the sibling rivalry phenomenon, child-teacher conflict, is followed by group discussion and suggestions on more appropriate ways of handling these problems. The reality testing that comes from being with the peer group allows perceptions of self and others to change. The substitute parental or other authoritative figures that the group therapists come to represent, allows the child the opportunity, within the safety of the group, to re-examine relationships with the adults in his own life. Other therapeutic factors relate to the small group dynamic that fosters a sense of responsibility and accountability of the group members towards each other, to the general framework of the group which comprises preset boundaries and limits, which presupposes therapist consistency, reliability and trustworthiness and offers suitable group composition to include children of both sexes or the same sex, of an age interval of no more than two years between them, and presenting with problems that are diverse but complementary. The therapeutic aim in group work, stated quite simply, is to help in the psycho-social readjustment of the children who are having difficulties in their group relationships.

In the past, groupwork has been largely nondirective, based on psycho-analytic thinking, practised only by those with such a training and offering mainly long term treatment contracts. We, the authors, would like to suggest that there is a strong case for bringing group therapy into line with other modern treatment approaches, and to stress its potential as an effective and economical way of helping large numbers of children over relatively short periods of time. Our own practice as illustrated in the latter half of this chapter, would suggest that the directive approach allows for the lifetime of the group to be structured in such a way as to meet the needs of the group that have been established at the outset. It also allows the kind of flexibility to cater for the newer and changing needs that invariably arise in the course of the treatment process. The work itself, we would suggest, is based in a theoretical framework that encompasses broad psychodynamic principles, an understanding of child development and an attention to sociological principles that govern everyday life. Clearly the intention here is to broaden the remit of group practice as well as group practitioner status to include all of those people, who work with children, who feel sufficiently competent and whose competence comes from a background of training and supervised experience, to take up the challenge of groupwork.

There now follows a summary of our observations of a particular group session that will, hopefully, illustrate our practice and orientation in working with groups of children.

A GROUP IN ACTION

Meeting No. 7

Three boys and two girls aged between nine and eleven years are in the waiting area with their parents. Dave and Jack are engaged in animated conversation. Paul is sitting close by his mother. Jane is reading a magazine, while Mary is looking around anxiously. The two therapists, one male one female, arrive at the appointed time and the children rush forward, down the corridor, ahead of the therapists and to the group room. They take off their coats and begin to explore the room. Mary does not as yet feel safe enough and keeps her coat on. It has been a week since the group last met and they have ahead of them an hour of group time. The group began meeting seven weeks ago and the future of the group life will be reviewed at the twenty week stage.

Last week the group had completed a mural that they had been painting in the previous six weeks, devoting the first twenty minutes of each session to this activity. Each member's contribution had been individual and thematic and had involved discussion about what they had produced. Today there would be no painting, something of a relief for the group members who sometimes found it difficult to talk about or to express their innermost feelings.

The first activity is the 'mime game'. All the group members, including the therapists, sit in a circle and a pencil is passed round in turn. The therapist starts by miming with the pencil the act of combing. Everyone shouts spontaneously 'comb' and the game begins. The first round is easy and everyone has ideas. Later the children begin consulting each other and producing helpful ideas for each other. Some take longer than others to produce a mime. The group becomes irritated with *Paul* who is a ditherer. He can be given half a dozen suggestions but is unable to make up his mind. Paul has great difficulties at school in terms of being accepted by his peers. He complains of being bullied and picked on. Mary, on the other hand, gets her turn done very quickly because she is too anxious to come up with her own ideas and acts immediately on any suggestion that is made for her. Mary comes from a materially and emotionally deprived background. She is lacking in confidence, enuretic and short-sighted. She is always eager to please, perhaps indiscriminately so. The mime activity lasts for about a quarter-of-an-hour. During this time the children have been sitting in a small and familiar circle and have been actively engaged with each other, thereby fostering a secure group cohesiveness. The therapists have provided for the group a model of greater tolerance towards its more needy members, who will, in turn, have derived some insight into their own difficulties from within the peer group.

The next activity is called the 'group interview'. It follows immediately on the previous one and the children have remained seated on the floor. A volunteer is called for who will answer questions from the other group members. The idea is to provide the children with the opportunity of learning more about each other. Clearly they will have some knowledge of each other from meeting in the previous few weeks. However, it is unlikely that they will have shared much personal or biographical information given the unwritten code of personal privacy. The therapists feel that the group has developed enough mutual trust to engage in this exercise. A volunteer emerges and the members take turns for both the asking of and answering questions. From an initial wondering about each others' material possessions, viz. toys, hobbies and interests, etc, the questions gently lead into asking about the family set up. *Dave* is able to tell the group with much evident relief that his parents are divorced and that he lives with his mother. Dave, an artistic and intelligent boy, has been referred primarily for temper tantrums in the home that had become worse following an episode in which he had witnessed his mother having sexual intercourse with her boyfriend on the lounge settee. Dave is unable to share this particular bit of information with the group. He knows that the group therapists know, but will not tell until he himself is able to trust the group enough to tell them himself. Other children exchange information about themselves and there is a feeling at the end of the exercise of knowing and perhaps even understanding each other.

In the above exercise a few, albeit significant, differences have been highlighted among the group members in terms of background, attitudes and presentation. It becomes important to avoid polarisation, or to reinforce extreme images of the self. A new activity is introduced that is called spectrum. An imaginary line is drawn across the room with the two ends representing extreme points of view. An example is given to the members, 'All those who like chips at one end of the room and all those who don't to the other end.' There is a rush to one end and no prizes for guessing which! The topics progress from non-threatening items to the family and personal issues. *Jack*, who is a skinhead and frequently in trouble for fighting in the classroom, has talked about the need to keep a macho image to stop others from bullying him. He says that he would love to be accepted by the peer group and implied that the reason he wasn't was because his peers did not think him good enough. When invited to rate himself along the spectrum of self-image ranging from good to very good, he placed himself with some difficulty at the good end of the pole, but with some encouragement from the group was able finally to stand at a point halfway between the two poles.

The final and brief exercise was a 'calming down' one which allowed the children to return to their parents in a reasonably happy state of mind.

At the end of the group the therapists met to discuss the structure and dynamics of the meeting. The above description gives some idea of the structure of the group. An example of the group dynamics may be found in the observations of *Jane's* behaviour, in her need to be the parental child, to help the 'mum' therapist to organise, to clean and tidy up and then to be the good one when the sibling members were in a squabbling mood. Jane, an obese girl had been referred for encopresis and difficulty in getting on with her father. The group response to her 'goodiness' was mildly resentful but not openly so and it was left to the therapist to look out in the future for competition among group members to try to gain therapist favours by similar 'good' behaviour, and in the event of its occurrence to make a suitable group interpretation.

2 Parents and toddlers need groups too!

The pre-school child population of Great Britain can be divided into two groups, namely the under-threes and those who are three-years of age and older. This arbitrary division is made on the basis of services available to the various groups of children. Thus, the older children have a variety of provisions made for them in terms of education and social services providing nursery schools, day nurseries, play groups, etc, while the younger group enjoy few, if any, of these facilities. The purpose of this chapter is to try to redress the balance of the need between these two groups of children.

The pre-school play group association (PPA), currently in its 25th year, proposed at its 1981 AGM that equal consideration be given in the future to the setting up of Parent and Toddler Groups (PT groups) by PPA branches in the counties and regions. By implication, the parents and toddler groups were to merit the same attention and consideration as has been the privilege of the pre-school play group in the past. Whether or not this proposal has come to fruition is a matter for examination of current practise and it could appear that the intervening six years since the proposal was first made has seen little movement in reaching the goals set at the time. For the purpose of clarification, the pre-school play group invites children of three years and above to join in their group activities. These children are regarded as being at a developmental stage where they can be safely separated from their parents for the duration of the group. Younger children on the other hand, are not felt to be ready for this experience and it is recommended that group activities for this age group should involve the children as well as their parents in a joint venture referred to in this chapter as the parent and toddler groups.

It is clear from the evidence in the literature as well as from a common-sense point of view, that pre-school children and their parents together form a sector of the population that has unique needs of its own. Younger parents of very young children within this group have even greater needs, not least those in terms of support and encouragement in their parenting roles. This may well be prefaced by the need for teaching and advising in parenting skills. After all, nobody is a born mother or a born father and, regardless of mythology, the maternal or parental instinct is never quite enough. There is a need for learning, shaping, recognising and tuning into the needs of the growing infant.

Much of this, unfortunately, is taken for granted and little allowance is made in many instances for inexperience, for lack of support within or outside the family, the lack of a confidante who can share in the feelings of joy or frustration of young parenthood or the numerous other factors that sometime conspire to add to the burden of care. Reference is being made here to illegitimacy, less of a stigma now than in the past, to single-parent families, to parents who feel socially isolated, who have personal difficulties, who may have housing and financial problems, and others in similar situations where the task of bringing up children is fraught with material, as well as emotional difficulties. Of course, there will be some parents who will be fortunate enough to have an extended family structure that is supportive in their endeavours. Parents might enjoy a warm and positive relationship with their own spouses, confiding in each other in times of stress. There will be some parents who will have the benefit of hindsight in being second, third or fourth timers or who have an opportunity to model on the good example of close friends and relatives. The point that is being made, however, is that even well placed parents need all the help that they can get to make a 'proper job' of bringing up a child that is in the end mutually satisfying to the parents, the child and the family.

The parent and toddler group does not pretend to provide all the answers to the questions that arise in the complex area of child-rearing. This clearly is the primary responsibility of the health, education and social services agencies who must adopt preventative as well as remedial measures to ensure the health and development of the children and the well-being of their parents. What the PT group does offer is the opportunity for parents to meet and mix, to exchange ideas and information on problem areas, to support and encourage each other in their tasks, to learn from the experiences of others and to model, where useful, on other parents' handling of their children. It also offers parents the opportunity to relax, chat, have a cup of tea without hurrying, make friends and widen their social circle. Opportunities may be available for guest speakers, health visitors, teachers, psychologists, social workers, doctors, to be invited to talk with the parents about various aspects of child development. For the child the PT group offers the opportunity of meeting and playing alongside or with other children of similar age and development in a happy and welcoming environment; to engage in structured or unstructured activities and for access to play materials that would not perhaps be available to them in their own homes; to feel safe in the knowledge that their parents will be present at all times to return to, to be comforted if distressed, to join in with their games if requested, or simply to be there to allow them the safety of a base from which to explore the new environment.

SETTING UP THE PARENT AND TODDLER GROUP

PT groups sometimes appear to arise from nowhere and then, like mushrooms spread geographically, flourish for a while and then disappear again. A chance television or radio programme on child-rearing may strike a chord with a few mothers living in the same area. A newly appointed health visitor brings in fresh ideas for helping the parents and children in her 'patch'. A local play group leader may recognise the needs of parents whose child attends the pre-school play group but have younger children at home whose needs are not being met. Similarly, social workers engaged with families in difficulties, community nurses, school teachers and other like-minded professionals, may decide or be prompted into a decision by some event or incident in their work with the families concerned, that there is a need for a local PT group that would in some way alleviate the problems with which they are working. The NSPCC officer for the area may feel that a PT group would be timely and useful in certain circumstances and thus would initiate setting up of such a group.

Thus there are a number of ways in which PT groups can get started and it is perhaps precisely because of this 'arising from need at the time' basis that the PT groups often assume an ephemeral quality. Here today, gone tomorrow. There is no tradition as such which allows for an open rolling group that can take on new members when old ones leave. Why this should be the case can perhaps be related to a curious twist of bureaucracy. Thus, because PT groups have parents as members of the group the laws relating to the Nursery and Childminders Regulations Act 1948, revised in 1968, do not apply. In other words, there is no statutory obligation on the part of Social Services, Education or Health Service agencies to provide, maintain or be responsible for the existence of such groups because the parents themselves are held to be responsible for the groups that they run. For once it would seem that the absence of red tape works against rather than in favour of the PT group.

Other reasons for PT groups folding up relate to practicalities such as children growing older, families moving on, professional workers finding other more pressing commitments and so on.

To end on a more optimistic note, however, it can safely be said that regardless of how a particular group becomes established, i.e., in terms of the needs identified at the time and the role of the people who initiated and maintained the project to its completion, the experience of participation in the group is invariably enriching and satisfying and the wish is that others should experience the same and that the group should continue for the benefit of those to follow.

Premises and Equipment

PT groups have been known to operate in a variety of settings. The local church hall or community centre often being the first choice for the group given their centralised position, the likelihood of the premises being available free of charge and the general feeling that the group represents a community activity and that the premises in question are there to serve the needs of the community. This does not, of course, preclude the search for other equally suitable accommodation and offers to use somebody's front room or basement, outhouse or garage, rooms in the local health service surgery or vacant space in a nearby school are quickly snapped up. The requirements as one would expect are for the place to be clean, warm and dry, to be available at specified times and to be cheap or free if possible. Fringe benefits would include the use of storage space, cupboards, store rooms and shelf space, cooking facilities or at least an area in which food and drink can be prepared. Other bonuses would include permission to modify the decor to make the environment as attractive and inviting as possible. Finally, it would be particularly helpful if there was more than one room available so that the parents have an opportunity to get together, relax, chat and so on. Prior to the actual use of the premises, it is important to establish some sort of agreement on how the premises are to be used and this will constitute a contract between the users and the landlord. In this, account will have to be taken of costs in terms of heating, insurance, etc, that are incurred in the running of the group.

As far as equipment is concerned the better provided the group is, the more stimulating and entertaining it becomes for its participants. This, of course, is easier said than done and we are immediately into the business of fund-raising from jumble sales, charity bazaars, raffles, sponsored activities, voluntary contributions and donations of used but intact toys and learning materials. In this connection, it is worth mentioning the Urban Aid Grant for inner-city areas that may come from Government sources of from the EEC, and for which projects such as the PT groups may well qualify. Once the money is collected, from whatever source, decisions have to be made on the choice of age appropriate play materials. A balance will be struck on the allocation of the limited funds to purchase equipment for messy play, for educational play materials, toys of various description and other items that have a regular turnover such as play-doh, powder paints, glue, paper, crayons, etc, as well as money for snacks, toiletries and other consumer items. The shopping list may seem endless but it is amazing how a little ingenuity and a lot of hard work can produce the goods on a shoe-string budget.

Having got the necessaries, the next step is in arranging the materials in such a way as to allow the children to identify different places within the room for different activities. Thus there will be a library corner, the home corner, the hospital area, the area for sand and water play, and of course the free play area that will be suitably equipped for the children to play in. The essence is in the creation of an identity and a spirit within the premises that the parents and child can affiliate with.

Activities

Listed below are some suggestions that could be used to form the basis for a much wider repertoire of activities for parents and children attending the group. These, of course, have to be taken account of in terms of what is available, the practicalities and, of course, the degree of tolerance!

SAND
An important piece of equipment for the children would be a sandpit. This is the age when children like to be involved with messy play and sand can fulfil this requirement. In this instance the sandpit will have to be large enough to hold a number of children. Equipment such as buckets, spades, plastic miniature garden tools, etc, should be readily available. Initially the parents will have to be involved to encourage the activity. This involvement could take two forms:
a) One adult may be prepared to tell a story which would incorporate sand into it, such as a trip to the sea-side, and the children's activities could then lead onto sandpies, castles, etc.
b) The children are encouraged to play in the sand under a common theme, such as hiding hands or feet in the sand or hiding objects.

WATER
Water play again is another way to be messy and the children will find this highly enjoyable. This will have to be a supervised activity if the environment is such that too much water could cause disaster. One idea would be to collect containers of different sizes and shapes. These

are filled with coloured water. Colour the water all different colours using a food dye. The children will enjoy pouring the water into different empty containers. It would be useful to encourage more group awareness by using the colours as a focal point for communication. This could be achieved by guessing the colours or mixing the colours. Further attention can be gained by adding small objects to the containers, stoppering them and shaking them. Flower petals and sand grains are particularly useful because they take time to settle to the bottom of the container.

CONCLUSIONS

1 Both sand and water play are tactile and messy. Consequently they fulfil the needs relating to the child's stage of development.
2 The children are using the same materials at the same time and therefore a group situation begins to develop. Children begin to be aware of the presence of others and have the opportunity to communicate.
3 Both for the parents and children, a learning situation develops. Parents who have difficulties in relating to their children will observe different ways of handling children. Children who have little or no contact with other children will begin to experience the early stages of communication and sharing.
4 Sand and water can easily be used in the home as a play material and hopefully some ideas can be taken from the PT group to home. If the experience is good the activities will be popular in the future.

BAKING

Watching and imitating parents is another way in which the child develops and under this premise good group activities can develop. One very obvious activity would be a baking session. Make up the dough by adding equal parts of salt to flour. This will make the dough hard when baked and it can then be painted. Encourage the children to sit around a table. In the centre of the table include small rolling pins, fancy biscuit cutters and other interesting shapes which will cut pastry. Firstly, demonstrate how to roll a piece of pastry and have the children copy. Of course, they will need help especially at the cutting stage, but do allow them the opportunity to try and do it themselves. It is important that if they are happy with their end result then the adult should be. Bake the shapes slowly in the oven until hard or if there is no oven allow them to dry out over night. The hard shapes will then provide a further group activity by painting them.

GARDENING
Another group activity which often happens at home is that of gardening. If the premises do not have an outdoor area an indoor garden can be enjoyable and made very simply. The use of water cress seeds, carrot tops placed in water and peas or beans placed on blotting paper are quick growing and interesting.

Obviously little fingers may find seeds difficult to deal with, but carrot tops or peas are sturdy and can survive handling. Again all the children should sit around the same table and work together with parental help. When all the seedlings are ready they should be placed together at a central point in the room thus enabling interest to be maintained and watering to occur.

CONCLUSIONS

1. Baking and gardening are adult activities which the children can copy and learn from. As in the previous activities, they are quite messy and tactile.
2. No new skills are needed by the parents.
3. The efforts put into flattening the dough will allow a release of energy and likewise of a garden plot was available outdoors. By channelling energy into a therapeutic activity, frustrations, tensions and anxieties can be reduced.
4. The children all work on the same activities and again a group situation develops (see previous conclusions).

SOMETHING FOR THE PARENTS

Catering for the needs of the children does not mean that the parents' own needs should be forgotten. Therefore, we would like to suggest some ways in making the parental contact a supportive network allowing a forum for discussion and ventilation.

One very obvious way is to get together with a cup of tea and maybe this form of contact will be all that is required for some parents. However, perhaps a definite weekly meeting with a particular focus may add more zest rather than it just being an exhausted recovery period from demanding children.

Soapbox Debate

Each person writes out a number of controversial issues on separate slips of paper. Each one is worded so that it can be answered by 'yes' or 'no'. For example, 'Should children be out of nappies by three years?' The group sits around in a circle and one person takes a slip of paper and reads it to the rest of the group. That person gives their opinion of 'yes' or 'no' and backs it up with two reasons. When the person has finished the topic is open for debate. Each group member should have a chance to take a slip of paper. Consequently the time taken over debating will relate to the number of people in the group.

CONCLUSIONS

1. Each person is allowed an opinion with the opportunity for expressing thoughts.
2. The topics chosen allow the opportunity to vent feelings over issues which may have been suppressed for various reasons, such as feelings of low self-esteem or feeling inadequate as a parent.
3. The group develops a way of communicating as a whole rather than one person being a spokesman, speaking for the more shy individuals.
4. To encourage a rise in self-esteem as each person will be listened to as a group.

ART ACTIVITY

Art is an excellent way to express oneself especially if verbal communication is not a strong point. Why not make use of the children's paints and use them for a parental group activity?

Paint a Topic

Each person writes out a topic which takes into consideration issues related to personal feelings, such as 'Children are demanding', or 'I need a holiday'. These are then mixed up and only one is taken and read out. Whatever is read out, each person will paint a picture of the topic incorporating their own feelings. At the end of the painting time each person shares their painting with a few comments about the meaning behind it. Usually discussion will emerge when questions are asked.

CONCLUSIONS

1 Art allows self-expression and is non-threatening because one is able to do one's own thing.
2 Although everybody is individual in their expression, everyone is doing the same thing so the self-conscious barriers drop.
3 The art focus allows the group to bring into the open topics which may be difficult to discuss in front of a larger audience.
4 Art can be relaxing after dealing with energetic children.

3 Stepping into the world of the nursery school

The first day at nursery is a landmark for the child and for the family. For the child this will be his first taste of the new world in which he will meet adults he has never met before and children with whom he has never played before. For the family the significance of the child's first day at nursery might lie, firstly, in the letting go of the child from the bosom of the family, secondly, in placing trust in the hands of those who will care for the child whilst he is away from home and, thirdly, in the acknowledgement that the child has taken his first step towards becoming, in time, a fully fledged member of society.

Nurseries may be run under the educational authorities when they are referred to as nursery schools, or by the social work authorities when they are referred to as social work day nurseries. Nurseries may be run privately or by voluntary agencies. Children are usually eligible to attend nursery at three years of age and until such time as the child become eligible to attend primary school. Social work day nurseries may take children of any age from a few weeks old to just under five years of age depending on the circumstances of the family concerned. The staffing arrangement varies in different nurseries and will consist of nursery nurses, teachers, social workers and auxiliaries. The input provided for the children will also vary from place to place and will depend on such factors as the staff–children ratio as well as the designation of the nursery as being an educational or social work responsibility. Perhaps the most important feature that determines the kind of experience that the child will receive during his stay is concerned with the ethos of the place, a term which is difficult to describe but which will include such things as the prevailing atmosphere, be this happy, stimulating, motivated or indifferent. The ethos itself will derive from the traditions set within the establishment in terms of child care, from good communications between the staff and from the kind of leadership provided by the administrative head of the nursery.

The provision of nursery facilities across the country is to say the least unevenly distributed with areas of the greatest need often being deprived of resources. This is not helped by the confusion that arises from different nurseries being accountable to different authorities, as a result of which, there seems to be a lack of cohesive policy or planning that takes account not only of the needs of the children but of the parents as well. Some regional councils in Britain are attempting to resolve this dilemma by including the provision of all services for the under-fives within the remit of one particular authority. Thus in the Strathclyde Region, for example, services for the under-fives including nursery schools, day nurseries, playgroups, chemists, playareas, health clinics, road crossings or provision in shops and restaurants are all being designated as the responsibility of one particular authority. In this instance, it is the educational authority that is to take responsibility for these services. The aim of the council is to involve the parents and other professionals in discussions as to the needs and type of services that should be provided for this age group.

The kind of scheme described above allows for opportunities to do preventive work that would not otherwise be easily available. A multi-disciplinary approach to child care is made possible where various professionals can meet and exchange ideas on the identified needs of the child and the family. Thus teachers, nurses, social workers, psychologists, psychiatrists, paediatricians, general practitioners and others can work together in assessing the child, identifying his needs and coming to some arrangement on how those needs can be met. In addition, for the child who is seen to be in difficulties at nursery or in the home and where it is clear that continued professional input will be necessary, the multidisciplinary approach will prove to be the ideal way of meeting these needs.

In the following paragraphs we shall be looking at some of the difficulties experienced by the child at nursery, and we will be looking at these difficulties under the headings of: away from home, the shy child, the distracting child and handling differences. A description of the difficulties will be followed by some suggestions for group exercises that might be of value in coping with these problems.

AWAY FROM HOME

For many children the initial few days at nursery will be their first experience of being away from home. Other children may have had the experience of being at Parent and toddler groups, although this will have been in the company of their parents. Going to nursery can therefore be a strange and exciting experience or, for that matter, a frightening experience for some children. There will be a new peer group and strange adults with whom the child will need to relate. In recognising these potential problems, most nurseries will allow for mothers or fathers to accompany their child and to stay with him on the premises for up to a week or longer depending on how soon it takes the child to settle in. Despite these precautions some children will continue to experience separation anxieties and will show distress when their parents leave. These anxieties may well be a manifestation of the child's own worries about being left alone in a strange environment although it may equally reflect separation difficulties on the part of the parents, particularly the first time parent. As far as the child is concerned, the problem may reflect the anxiety of being abandoned or rejected, or the fear of being unable to cope within the new environment. These problems in turn may reflect the lack of a secure attachment or result from a kind of social isolation in which the child is quite simply unable to make the transition from the close nuclear family to the hustle and bustle of the nursery.

The kind of distress shown in these children will consist of such behaviours as crying spells, inability to settle, clinging behaviour, regressive behaviour including incontinence, and a refusal to take part in structured activities.

The following exercise is quite a simple activity which harks back to infancy and in which the child engages repeatedly in building brick towers and then knocking them down.

Building Towers

A large number of various sized building bricks are required. Bright and colourful ones will be more appealing. The activity is set up in a central position so that the 'new' children are aware of what is happening. The group worker encourages the children to build towers as high as possible until they fall down. Children enjoy watching the towers fall and enjoy even more in knocking them down. Providing no demands are made on the 'new' children, they will find it difficult to resist becoming involved, even if this is only in watching and not actually joining in.

18 CHILDREN NEED GROUPS

CONCLUSIONS

1. The task offers a non-threatening structure, is not demanding and therefore it is not creating further anxiety.
2. The task is one which is familiar and used throughout childhood. Therefore, it is comforting in this new environment.
3. Any child can participate when they are ready.
4. The brightness and the physical activity will provide a focus which will detract from the strange situation they have found themselves in.
5. The activity can be part of an introductory repertoire of games for a new intake of children or can be specially 'arranged' to help out the child who is new to the group.

THE SHY CHILD

Some children seem to lack the confidence or self-assuredness to interact in a mutually satisfying way with their peer group. There are obviously many reasons for this kind of situation developing, and these would range from the child who is unable to interact with his peers because he has a very low self-esteem, to the child who is unable to do so because he has never had the experience of having done so in the past. The children may be inhibited from communicating with others because they are unable to do so adequately in that they have difficulties either in speech or in some comprehension. A child may not be as physically robust as the rest of the children or actually have motor or neurological problems. The child may come from a family that is socially isolated and where there is little by way of modelling from the rest of the family in the social sense. The shy child is often a lonely child and adults who recognise this in the nursery may well seek to fill in the gaps themselves when perhaps it would be in the child's best interests for the child to receive encouragement to actually interact with his own peer group. Also it is known that by the age of three, children engage in co-operative play rather than merely playing alongside each other at the more infant level and it would be useful to deploy this natural developmental phase to encourage the child to participate in activities by providing the kind of structured games that are enjoyable learning experiences. The shy child is easily enough recognised in his hanging back from the rest of the group, and preferring to engage in solitary activities while at the same time clearly indicating at all times that probably if things were better in himself he would wish to be with the rest of the group.

This group exercise is designed to provide the child with an opportunity, 'under cover' as it were, to become actively involved with the peer group.

The Use of Puppets

In most areas of a nursery there is a corner which is suitable to house a puppet theatre. In fact, in one nursery we visited we were delighted to find a small area made into a mini-theatre. Puppets come in all shapes and sizes and portray all kinds of characters. They are very useful, therefore, for encouraging children to become more expressive and involved without feeling self-conscious about it.

Supply a good selection of hand puppets and ask the children to select one or two puppets. Hand puppets are easily manipulated at any nursery age level. When all the children have at least one puppet, sit with the children and help them to start a story which will include the puppets. This need only be short, because once the puppets are in the children's hands there is usually an eagerness to start using them. Encourage the puppet play to begin, directing only when there is a need. If the story line to the adult is somewhat difficult to understand this will be of little importance if all the children are able to become involved and look like they are enjoying the experience. An added incentive for the children to put on a really good show could be had by way of providing an appreciative audience.

CONCLUSIONS

1 To be able to hide behind a puppet will help the child to forget his/her shyness and therefore begin to interact constructively with the peer group.
2 Positive encouragement from the players will help to increase a child's self esteem.
3 The social structure of the play will create a useful modelling experience, e.g. turn taking, etc.
4 For children with verbal communication problems the puppet can say as little or as much as he likes.
5 Having an appreciative audience will help the child to feel part of both the performing as well as the wider group, and in this way help create a sense of belonging.

THE DISTRACTING CHILD

Some children, instantly recognisable, seem to be more of a handful for nursery staff than others. These children are described as being or seeming to be constantly 'on the go'. They seem to have more energy than the others, are less willing or able to tend to one task at a time, and during free play are found as likely as not to be interfering with other children's activities causing a degree of disruption. Again as with the shy child there are many reasons for this kind of behaviour, so that the label often applied to these children of 'the hyperactive child' can be both misleading and inaccurate. Clearly there are clinically hyperactive children whose pervasive pathological behaviour leaves no doubt as to the diagnosis. The distracting child, on the other hand, manifests behaviours, the causes of which are to be found mainly in the psycho-social factors rather than in constitutional factors. Thus the behaviour described could be attributed to high levels of anxiety, understimulation of the child in the home environment, the child coming from a large family, inadequate modelling for the child on what is acceptable and what is not and in terms of limit setting on certain kinds of behaviour in the home.

Attending the nursery provides the child with the kind of opportunity where he can learn to interact more appropriately with his peer group as well as with the adults who look after him. Where facilities are available for a multidisciplinary approach to this kind of problem then it is possible to involve the parents and the family of the child in looking at how the overall situation might be helped.

The following group exercise requires the child to express himself constructively through sound and action.

Use of Music

Before the session collect a variety of percussion instruments, some ready made and others that have been made by the children as a group activity. Thus, for example, putting dried pulses into cartons, yoghurt pots or boxes and sealing the containers. These end up in all shapes and sizes, in different colours and producing different sounds.

Begin the session by encouraging each child to sit in a circle and allowing them to choose one instrument. Using a record-player or cassette-player select a piece of music with which the children are familiar, i.e., a nursery song or a pop song. Explain to the children that when the music begins they will play their instruments to the music they hear. This can happen with all the children playing together, accompanying the music, each in turn, trying out each others percussion boxes and listening to various kinds of music.

CONCLUSIONS

1 Music (sound and action) allows for the expression of energy and drive particularly useful for the distracting child.
2 The activity offers a structure but, at the same time, freedom of expression.
3 All the children are involved in the same task, therefore producing a social learning experience.
4 Verbal skills are not called upon and only minimal developmental skills are required to participate in this activity.

HANDLING DIFFERENCES

For many children the experience of attending nursery comes as something of a surprise in terms of what is expected of them in this new environment. Thus they will be expected to sit in a group, to wait their turn, to participate in structured activities and to learn how to get on in this new mini society. Above all the child learns that he is just one of a group of children and that his needs and wants do not take precedence over that of the others. He also learns that the adults are there to give of themselves, to look after him and to have their own expectations of his giving something in return.

One of the problems encountered by staff and parents of children attending the nursery is that of reported discrepancies in behaviour between home and nursery. Thus parents may report difficulties with the child at home which are not manifest while the child is at nursery or vice versa. Thus the model child at nursery might be said to behave like a tyrant at home while in other cases the opposite may apply. Invariably these problems can be attributed to differences in style of handling between parents and the nursery staff. Clearly there are many reasons why this may be so but what tends to happen at times is that parents and staff in these instances can become highly critical of each other. The resulting atmosphere is obviously not in the child's best interests in terms of his future growth and development and one way of rectifying this kind of situation is where parents and staff can meet regularly to discuss the progress of their particular child. This may take the form of formal or informal meetings between parents and staff or what would be much more useful would be in terms of parents actually attending the nursery at regular intervals and taking part in structured activities along with the staff.

The following group exercise involving parents, staff and children may help to avoid this kind of conflict arising. It utilises art as a particularly effective way of engaging the young child and his parents in joint activity.

Art Activity

A good supply of art materials will be required including suitable items to enable a collage to develop. Ask the group to work on their own piece of paper following a theme. The theme can be chosen in relation to something appropriate to the nursery, home or the time of year. Explain that there will be at least twenty minutes to work on the theme and produce a picture. At the end of the time all the pictures can be viewed by everyone and better still put onto the wall.

CONCLUSIONS

1 With staff and parents working together with the children a joint sense of responsibility is fostered for the group as a whole.
2 Children will find added security in seeing their parents participating along with other parents and staff in a group activity.
3 An opportunity is provided for parents to model on each other and staff in dealing with their children during the minor altercations that inevitably occur in such activities.
4 An awareness is created on how children may interact differently with different adults and this can be used for later informal and friendly discussion with the adult group.

ADDITIONAL EXERCISES

There are many musical exercises to consider and they are particularly useful as a group activity. Listed below are some games that seem eternally popular and of the type that children seem rarely to tire of.

Musical Games

A tape-recorder or record-player is required to supply the music. Use music which is familiar to the children. Pop music will do nicely!

STEPPING INTO THE WORLD OF THE NURSERY SCHOOL

1 **STATUES**
The children are asked to dance about to the music, but when the music stops they must freeze into a statue. If they move they are out. If and when they are out it is *important* to give the child a task such as helping with the music or watching for other children to move. This will prevent boredom and distractability and give the child a sense of responsibility.

2 **MUSICAL BUMPS**
Again the children dance about until the music stops. As soon as this happens they must sit on the floor. The last one down is out. After sitting out for two times the child is allowed back in. The exercise stops when the children are exhausted.

3 **MUSICAL CHAIRS**
Chairs are set out in the middle of the room with one less chair than the number of children. The children move round and round the chairs until the music stops. When the music stops the aim is to sit on a chair. The one child who does not have a chair is out and becomes a helper to the leader. Each time one chair is removed until only one chair remains and two children are left to try to sit on the chair.

CONCLUSION

1 Music and movement is a good means of expression. It releases tension and is relaxing.
2 The music and the activity described will be familiar and therefore non-threatening. The activity itself is vigorous with a competitive edge and this seems to concentrate the mind wonderfully! (see the distracting child).
3 The activities are rule bound and constitute the beginnings of socialisation and group interaction.

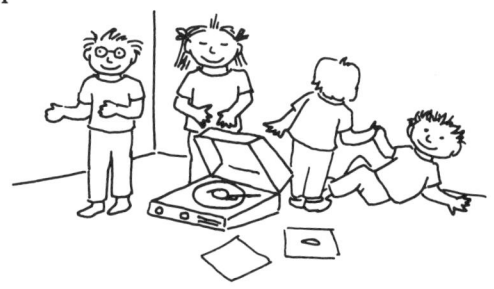

4 How do I look?

'Know Thyself' is a common dictum. It is particularly true of those engaged in the caring profession. The question is, how many of us can really claim to 'know' ourselves? What do we physically look like to other people? How do we come across in social situations? What characteristic emotions and feelings do we respond with, to situations and people? What kind of intellectual capacities or talents do we possess? Most importantly, how does self perception match the image that others may have of us? These are difficult questions that may remain unanswered in a lifetime. Perhaps ignorance is bliss! Maybe we do not feel the need to consciously set about thinking and answering these questions. It is possible that the whole process is preconscious and that over time we learn to modify, adapt to and change according to the demands of circumstances. In short we learn by trial and error to present the acceptable parts of ourselves and equally to hide the less pleasant bits. With children however this process of living and learning about themselves is as yet fresh, new and exciting by sheer virtue of their age and limited experience of life. Even so it is possible to experience within this short space of time the sort of traumas that make the child mistrustful, resentful and bitter in relationships with adults and other children. These feelings are usually prompted by a basic notion of unworthiness and low self-opinion.

In this chapter we shall be looking at anomalies and oddities of physical appearance that may give cause for the child to develop a poor opinion of himself. In this context we shall consider facial characteristics, gestures and mannerisms, speech and physique of the child. We shall also look at the problems faced by the coloured child and look briefly at the area of physical handicap—a subject that will be covered more fully in a subsequent chapter. Group exercises are described to include the aim or purpose of the exercise, the method to be used and the ways in which we feel that the exercise might be useful for specific problems found by the child. Where possible brief descriptions of clinical cases may be used to illustrate the point.

HOW DO I LOOK? 25

FACIAL CHARACTERISTICS

Children are quick to pick up and then sometimes target special features about other children (and adults). Nicknames are a common feature of school life and much as they are uncalled for, frequently represent accurate descriptions of the person being nicknamed with regard to some aspect or other of personality or presentation. The child with a large nose, the one with ears that stick out, the child wearing glasses, the child with bad teeth, with a skin condition, with badly cut hair and a host of other minor blemishes will become ready targets for teasing and name calling. These children may react to this in a variety of ways. More commonly they may just put up with it. Some will put up a fight and depending on their size and personality may well succeed in getting away with it. Others might join in the game and themselves select names for other children. With the exception of the third type of child the first two categories of children will invariably suffer. Having said this, however, the point that needs to be made at this time is that discrete or isolated causes for complaint are rarely by themselves the reason for general unhappiness. More often than not there are a cluster of items that together form the basis for a troubled sense of being. We shall consider now ways of helping resolve some of these problems in the group exercise to be described.

EXERCISE 1

Self Portrait

The purpose of this exercise is in the first instance to emphasise similarities between individuals. This makes it possible for the group to feel secure enough to be able to look at the differences that exist between them. The emphasis at all times is on the enjoyment of the task.

METHOD
Ask the children to sit in a circle and provide various drawing materials. The children should begin the self portrait by putting their name on the paper, thus committing themselves to the task. It may be necessary to give ideas such as the therapist starting first, suggesting particular facial features and expressions or giving clues to their own physique. Allow about 10–15 minutes to complete the picture. On completion of each child's picture all the pictures should be accessible for each group member to see.

26 CHILDREN NEED GROUPS

To encourage some group discussion invite each child to say a few words about their portrait.

CONCLUSIONS

1. The picture rather than the child becomes the focus for discussion.
2. Since there are several pictures to be looked at, the focus becomes diluted further.
3. The group feedback allows for positive as well as critical remarks to be made.
4. This is made possible in the relaxed and safe atmosphere created by the therapist.
5. The therapist will know how much each of the children is willing or able to express themselves to the group.
6. The foremost message that the child takes away is the realisation of being very like his peers.

GESTURES AND MANNERISMS

These can often in later life be the hallmark of the personality. Mimics and cartoonists make their living by portraying gestures and mannerisms of the rich and famous. Not so for children the delights of being associated with nose picking or ear lobe tugging or shoulder twitching or head bobbing or the peculiarity of gait. Given that there are some who believe that mannerisms are actually inherited and others who believe in the modelling or imitative or habitual nature of the problem, it is in the end the sheer almost unhelpability and unawareness of doing it whilst doing it that makes the idiosyncratic gesture so easy to identify and abuse. Let us consider how the following exercise may be useful:

EXERCISE 2

Be Me

The purpose of this exercise is to learn by imitation. The child develops an empathetic understanding of what it feels like to 'be' someone else and equally learns by observation how he comes across to other people.

HOW DO I LOOK? 27

METHOD
The children are asked to find a partner. Each partner is given a small task to do such as explaining how to get from the 'group room' to the outside door. One person within the partnership will be the facilitator and the other person who is the receiver must copy all the facilitators movements. After a short time set another task for the other partner to do and follow the same procedure. Give some time for discussion and then move onto the next part if appropriate. If discussion is difficult ask each group member to say one thing they learnt about their own gestures or mannerisms.

The next part is to bring everyone together into a circle. Each individual in turn walks around the inner circle and consequently the circle starts to move round with the individual, again, copying their movements. Encourage positive comments on their walk/body posture which are based on observation.

Again allow time for discussion. With both exercises the therapists must be aware of any unsupportive comments or actions and deal with these appropriately. The child should leave the group feeling positive about himself/herself and not feeling they have been ridiculed.

By talking about David we may help to illustrate more about the exercise. David is rather a fat boy, who's clothes never look like they fit him properly. A usual feature is his trousers falling down from the waist to his hips. His social skills are not very good and he appears awkward in his movements. When we did this exercise with David it was difficult for David to believe the way he presented himself. The other children were not too sensitive towards him and it took a lot of work on our part to help him feel comfortable. We decided it would be more appropriate to work only in partners, rather than have David exposed to the whole group at once.

CONCLUSIONS

1 The initial painting of the children serves its own purpose of reducing isolation and encouraging interaction.
2 The use of non threatening activity puts the child at ease.
3 The act of imitating produces fun and laughter.
4 The children, in this context can then feel free to comment on each others actions.
5 If a sufficient amount of trust has developed within the group and if the children are feeling sufficiently confident then the second part

of the exercise can be used to compliment the first on the same or at a subsequent meeting.
6 The children go away feeling positively framed rather than embarrassed or ridiculed.

SPEECH

Speech delay, poor articulation, mumbling and stuttering all predispose to being poorly understood, underestimated, shunned, spoken loudly to as with the hard of hearing, easily lost patience with or generally made fun of and left out. For the child with the problem the frustration of being unable to communicate is devastating. There is inevitably a price to pay. Where language is all important these children are going to be singled out. No escape here to the woodwork class. Poor school performance, poor peer relationships are not uncommon. Coping is by fighting, aggression, poor concentration, distractibility, clowning, conduct problems at home and at school, or, on the reverse side of the coin, withdrawal, apathy, sadness and a feeling of the uselessness of trying. Low self opinion is at the core, resentment and anger the feeling that is either externalised inappropriately or turned in on the self. Sublimation is more the exception than the rule. Again as mentioned previously it is not the isolated symptom as much as the cluster that produces the clinical picture. This is especially so with problems of speech which can be accompanied by other developmental delays both motor and sensory. The following exercise may prove helpful where one or more children in the group have some form of speech difficulty.

EXERCISE 3

Story Wheel

The idea in this exercise is to encourage speaking without making the child self-conscious. The task is so constructed as to take away from it appearing to focus on speech and to shift attention from the non-verbal uses associated with speech difficulties.

METHOD
Ask the children to lie on their backs with their heads coming together in the centre and their legs forming an outer circle. Eyes closed. The children are told they are going to make up a story going around in a

circle. The story can be about anything and each child can say as much or as little as they like. It is useful if the therapist starts the story and brings it to a close at a convenient place. When the person feels they have said enough the story is passed onto the next person and so on. At the end of the story ask the children to sit up slowly, and think about events which happened in the story. A short discussion will round off the exercise.

CONCLUSIONS

1 The novelty of the arrangement creates a sense of anticipation.
2 Proximity to each other makes for a sense of security.
3 The Speech form becomes less important than the content in terms of the story that is being told.
4 Material from the story is illuminating of both the individual and the group thought process.

PHYSIQUE

Like the Good the Bad and the Ugly there is the tall the short the fat and the skinny. There is also the clumsy, the gawky, the butter-fingered. The one who is no good at sports or gym. These are the children who stand out from their peers. They stand out in a way that is inferior to the others. They know it and everybody else knows it and they have to compensate for it. It is an asset to be reasonably tall as an adult. It is fashionable to be skinny. The tall child is at risk of both looking and being made to feel different. If the skinny man gets sand kicked in his face on the beach then the equivalent happens to children who are perceived as weak and helpless by virtue of being underweight or thin. The short child is patronised and condescended to. The fat child is literally the Billy Bunter of the class. It is common knowledge that children who are good at sports and all things athletic are popular and well liked by their peers. The child who is averagely interested in sporting activities will get by. It is the child who has an aversion to matters physical who is at risk of being castigated by his peers: the awkward child is frequently the butt of jokes. The moral would seem to be simply that the child who is not of average size, build and co-ordination is at risk of having difficulties and this needs to be understood. The next exercise to be described is designed to help with some of these problems.

EXERCISE 4

Change of dress

The aim in this exercise is to pose an observational challenge to the members of the group. Paradoxically the challenge is to note changes in the external appearance, i.e. the dress of the challenger to the point where his physique becomes of secondary importance. Having fun is the operative term.

METHOD

The group form a circle. A volunteer is asked for and that particular member has to stand within the circle and slowly turn around. If a volunteer is not forthcoming the therapist may have to go first and be a model for the children. Each group member makes a mental observation about the volunteer. The volunteer goes out of the room and makes a subtle change to his/her appearance. Having done so he/she returns to the room and again physically displays themself. The other children in the group spend time guessing what the change could be.

Peter

Peter, a very bright, intelligent boy aged 11, had poor peer relationships. He found it difficult to use his peer groups language and actions. Someone observing the group said he was like a 'middle class, eccentric university lecturer'.

When we started to play 'Change of Dress' Peter appeared gangly and awkward when the attention was focused on himself. However the more it was played the more he began to relax and gain encouragement from the other children. He was also quick to notice changes when he was guessing things about the others. This allowed his intelligence to be used on the same level as the other children, without appearing the one who is good at 'school subjects'.

The following week when we met with the children Peter was the one who asked to play the game again.

CONCLUSIONS

1 The element of the 'game' is important in that it detracts from the child's preoccupation or self-consciousness regarding his physique.
2 The group members are subtly persuaded that it is not the physical

appearance of the child that is of concern as much as how clever he is or how quick they are in spotting the change of dress.
3 The comradeship that develops helps with familiarisation and a feeling of trust.
4 The exercise can indeed provide the child with an opportunity to show how creative or inventive he can be.

PHYSICAL HANDICAP

Included in this category are those children who suffer from congenital physical disability as well as those who suffer from chronic physical illness. The reason for considering these two groups of children is that they have in common 'real' physical problems. These may be handicapping in a variety of ways of minor facial deformities to major physical disability. In discussing these issues it is difficult to separate family influences and environmental factors that will obviously play a crucial part in helping, or for that matter hindering, the child's development. In fact most of the literature seems to emphasise these two aspects. Clearly these are important and will be discussed under appropriate headings in subsequent chapters. What is essential as far as the concept of physical awareness is concerned is the need to recognise the primary disability and the demands it places on the child in coping with the everyday hurly burly of life. The disability is in the first instance part and parcel of the child's physical being. The child may have irrational feelings of being somehow personally responsible for the condition. The burden of shame has to be carried because one is not as perfect as one's brother or sister or even the child next door. The feelings of rage at being singled out must inevitably be repressed if life is to remain enjoyable. There must be adaptation. The current educational provision takes account of the needs of these special groups and provides separate schools for the physically disabled, the chronically physically ill child who has lost time through repeated hospital admissions, for the delicate child, and can even provide home tuition under special circumstances. It is possible that the facilities for these children will be withdrawn in favour of 'all-in-one' schooling as a means towards promoting integration and reducing discrimination. The feasibility of such a move is debatable. Do these children, for example, prefer the company of similarly affected youngsters. Would they rather be in a 'normal' school. How do children without disability react to those with disability. Is it true that 'normal' children accommodate and are empathic towards children with disability. Does the same apply to these children in the community. We are assuming here that the one place where they are accepted fully is in their own homes and families. Perhaps it is all too easy to make this assumption. Maybe we should be asking the children for their views and opinions instead of making assumptions. We are talking here about children suffering from a range of conditions as diverse as hare lip and cleft palate, port wine stains, ptosis, hydrocephalus, facial asymmetries to congenital hemi and paraplegias, spina bifida congenital and acquired conditions cystic fibrosis, renal diseases requiring transplants and/or haemodialysis, diabetes, leukaemias. The list is endless. The following exercise may prove useful when one or more children in the group has some form of physical handicap.

EXERCISE 5

Draw round me

The aim of this exercise is to make group members aware of their physical boundaries, the personal space they occupy and to relate this to the physical and personal space of others around them. To become accepting and accommodating of others shape and form.

METHOD

For the exercise large sheets of paper are required (the reverse side of wallpaper can be used) plus pencil, felt tipped pens and paints. Each child must find a partner to work with. The paper is placed on the floor and one child lies on top of the paper, whilst the other child draws around him. When the drawing is complete the process is reversed. Next follows time for each individual to fill in their drawing with physical characteristics plus their clothing. Encourage the children to ask each other about themselves. A full length mirror placed in the room may be of help to the child who is too self conscious to ask others about their physical appearance. At the end of their art work pin each full life drawing up on the wall, so that the room is surrounded by a picture gallery of the group. Take time to view the pictures together as a group. It may be necessary at this point for the therapists to verbally make suggestions about the pictures, allowing a licence for others to do so.

John

John is a child who throughout his short life has been in and out of hospital with renal problems. He is twelve years old, very short and stocky built and has a very round 'moon' shaped face from taking steroids. Overall he looks older than his years, with an adult, self-assured attitude. He came to the group after a renal transplant, but before he joined us we were aware that he had problems with his body image. His drawings clearly indicated this (see fig. 1) as well as being sensitive over physique.

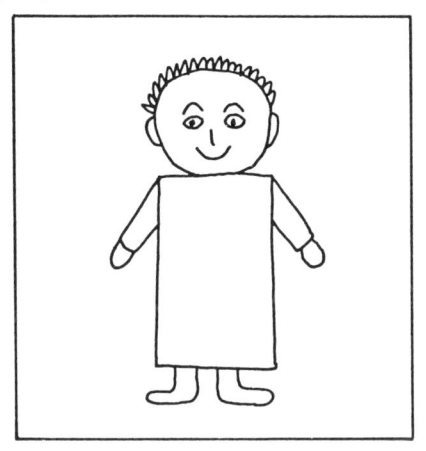

Fig. 1
Note: no neck, small fat body, short arms and legs, always a happy face.

We felt the exercise 'Draw round me' would help John to realise his own body shape and encourage him to feel more comfortable with himself. Within weeks John had modified his drawings of people (see fig. 2). He had also started to diet successfully. We would like to think 'Draw round me' and other exercises were a contributing factor to John's changed attitude.

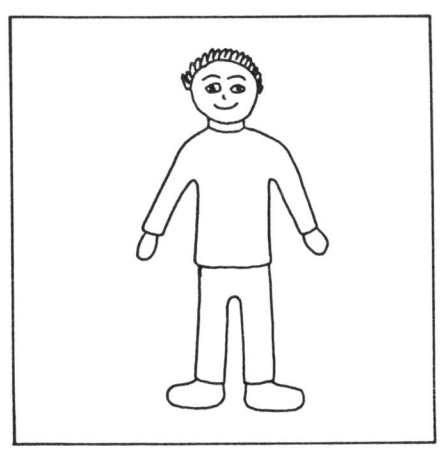

Fig. 2

CONCLUSIONS

1 This exercise is time consuming and absorbing and attracts full participation as a group activity.
2 The act of tracing the body outline provides a personal touch and creates a sense of closeness.
3 Often the completed figure is in many ways an accurate representation of the child which may then be seen and examined.
4 Deformities or distortions can be looked at matter of factly and children will develop a sympathetic attitude to those with such problems.

THE COLOURED CHILD

The preceding paragraphs have all stressed the point that to be out of the norm is to be at risk of difficulties. The same would very obviously apply to the child whose appearance does not tally with the rest of the group. The coloured child is particularly at risk here either of being actively excluded or, in seeking to identify with a fellow group of foreign children, of socially isolating himself. Alternatively he or she may join the host group denying their own origins and cultures with resultant conflict both within the child and with the family. In areas of high immigrant populations it is easier for the child to identify with children from the same background. Where this is not the case the child will have greater difficulties in adapting. It is interesting to note in this context that given the choice foreign children, i.e. coloured children, preferred to be seen as white or in any event of the same appearance as the host population. The problems that the coloured child encounters are once again those that he must have to cope with himself albeit with help from his family. Whether or not he does so successfully, the effort as in all other cases of deviation from the norm, is great and requires the support and understanding of all those in position to offer it. The following exercise can be used to help integrate the coloured child with the rest of the group.

EXERCISE 6

The Group Tangle

The aim of this exercise is to reduce the sense of social isolation experi-

HOW DO I LOOK? 35

enced by the coloured child. The physical and psychological distancing involved in social isolation can hopefully be bridged by this or similar exercises.

METHOD
One child volunteers to be the person who will eventually untangle the group. He sits with his back to the group therefore not looking at the way in which the tangle has evolved. The other members join hands in a circle leaving two ends of the circle open. The people at the ends of the circle become leaders and the interweaving and generally tangling all the group up. No-one must let go of hands or untangling becomes difficult. When the tangle is complete it is the volunteers job to try to return the tangle to its original state. The group can decide beforehand if the volunteer can physically move the tangled group about or if he is only to use language. Each person should be allowed to be the untangler and the leader of the tangle.

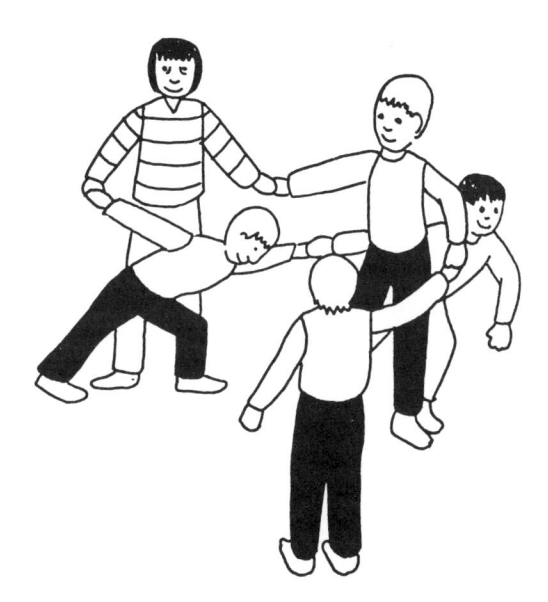

CONCLUSIONS

1 This exercise offers a lot of physical contact.
2 Group members have to be actively manipulated to form a tangle.

3   A feeling of group warmth and cohesiveness develops quickly.
4   A group identity forms at the expense of individual space so that each child (and therapist) is now a part of the chain and not seen to be coloured or in any way different from the rest of the group.

ADDITIONAL EXERCISES

Code
A   Physical awareness
B   Facial characteristics
C   Gestures and mannerisms
D   Speech
E   Physique/physical handicap
F   Coloured child

FACE, POSTURE AND MOVEMENT

The group is expected to move around for this exercise, which demands physical expression with an emotional content. The exercise can take various forms:

1   Ask the children to express how they are feeling today both facially and bodily. The children could guess each others movements, thus encouraging active participation.
2   Ask the children to move around in various ways depicting different emotions (happiness, sadness, anger, surprise, pain, etc).
3   Ask one child to mould another child in a posture of how that child appears.
4   Ask one child to mould all the other children into a group picture of how that child is feeling. Each child should be allowed a turn to do this.

These exercises will be particularly useful for exploring A, B, C, E, F.

Who Am I?

This exercise takes the form of a collage. It does not involve direct social interaction which can be useful if the children do not know each other well. Often sharing equipment such as paints, glue, etc, will help to break down social barriers.

METHOD
Ask the children to look through magazines and find pictures and words which would be descriptive of themselves. Suggest to the children they make a collage using pictures and words representing themselves. Allow time for discussion and sharing their work. The therapist will

HOW DO I LOOK? 37

need to be supportive to those children who have been able to expose themselves far more than the other children.

This exercise will help by exploring further all aspects of self-awareness.

Personal Object

This exercise is carried out with the children in a circle. This is a verbal exercise.

METHOD

Ask the children to think of an object which they possess. The children are then encouraged to become that object and to speak in the first person to describe the object. If this is too verbally demanding for a child they could be asked to think of one quality the object possesses. Allow the children time for spontaneous questions which will help the child to gain some feedback.

This exercise will be of particular help in exploring all aspects of self-awareness. Because the child is focusing on the object rather than themselves they will probably say more about themselves, thus highlighting the areas of self-awareness we have mentioned.

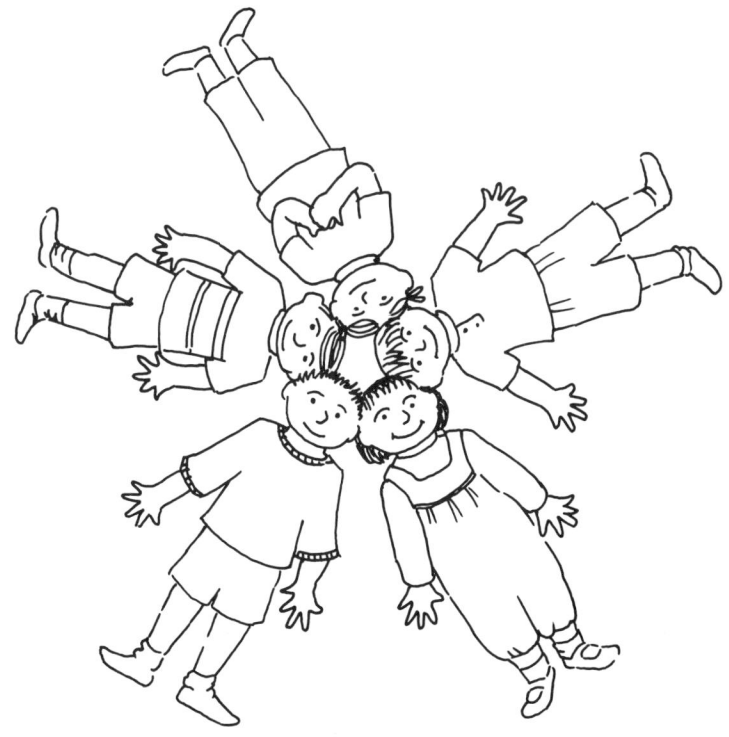

5 Society invites you to join its ranks

Every social group has its own misfit. This is usually achieved by a process of nomination. Thus, although the members of a particular group may complain bitterly about the errant member and are always thinking of ways to get rid of him, they never actually get around to doing so because every group needs its own misfit to serve the hidden purposes of the group. An alternative arrangement is where the position of the misfit is a rotating one. Here a process of self selection occurs or the group nominates a member for the particular occasion. The entire process is unconscious just as the purpose and needs of the group served by the misfit remain unconscious or at least not openly acknowledged. An illustration of this process is to be found for example at the cocktail party where there will be invariably the boorish, drunken, disorderly character who is seen to 'spoil' it for everybody else. What is amazing is that given the care with which guest lists are made up for such occasions how does one explain the regularity with which the 'spoiler' is invited. Perhaps the reason simply is to reassure everybody else about their own civility, niceness and social acceptability. Besides why indulge one's own need to misbehave on these occasions when somebody else is already doing it for you! Among children too there are the misfits, the conformists and those who sometimes fit and those who do not. It needs to be said at this point that there are a variety of factors that influence one's place and acceptability in society. When sociologists refer to the tribal nature of the society in which we live, there is a good-natured acceptance of it in much the same way as one would appreciate a good joke. When the Sunday papers attempt to explain football hooliganism in these terms it makes for interesting conversation. The fact is that references to tribes and tribal rites and customs evoke images of primitive and barbaric lifestyles which are best confined to the jungle of Borneo. The truth is that these rites and customs in essence prevail across cultures and civilisations and need to be understood in order to make sense of the social morals of our own times.

When we refer to a specific problem, such as little Johnny was an absolute angel until he started school or wee Lisa is the model pupil at school but a right little Hitler at home, then we move into the realms of society's norms, the demands it places on its members to conform to these norms and the sanctions it imposes for the violation of its dictates.

Social awareness then is the realisation of what is acceptable and what is not acceptable in terms of living with other people be this at school or at work, at home or in the community.

In the next few paragraphs we shall be looking at various aspects of the individual and the way in which he or she presents to and interacts with the outside world. This will then be followed by a sample of group exercises designed to promote social awareness and social skills, together with an understanding of the group dynamics involved.

SOCIABILITY

Primitive tribal customs, rites and rituals are never more prominent than with children, be they from the most 'civilised' of western societies. The child who refuses to recognise this structure or for some reason remains unaware of it will be the outcast, that is, until he is able to see the error of his ways, make suitable reparation and be re-initiated into the fold. If this sounds alien then let us start by looking at one aspect of adult life that has its parallels with the society of children. We have our hierarchical structures and nobody escapes them. The children have a more obvious pecking order. Promotion up the ladder in the first instance is by dint of age, size and brute strength. Animal cunning helps this process along in the context of the boss man dictating while the others listen. Each group has a boss man and his followers who are kept in line by the aid of the boss's henchmen. Several groups coexist, for the greater part, peacefully because there is mutual respect for each other and for each others code of practice and their territory. The child who does not 'get on' is basically refusing to accept the natural hierarchy. If he goes on to fight he is challenging the leadership of the hierarchy, which he is foolish to do unless there is support on the ground for change. In the absence of such support he is seen to be upsetting the natural rhythm of life. It therefore seldom becomes necessary for the leader to counter this challenge. He can safely leave this task to his followers, who will make sure that there is no infraction of the rules. The child thus becomes the one 'nobody wants to play with'. We may wonder why any child would wish to violate their society's code. A number of reasons can be postulated, some of which have already been dealt with in previous paragraphs. Perhaps the one common theme that pervades is that of the feeling of unfairness, of injustice from which these children who are said 'not to get along' seem to suffer. They are constantly striving to establish a sense of worth, in constant search of the feeling that they too are worth knowing. It is unfortunate that in their attempts to be recognised they pay little heed to the prevalent social custom and because of this are rejected by their peers.

To help the children establish a sense of their own worth they must first of all be encouraged to recognise their own position in the social hierarchy; once they have gained some awareness of this they can build upon both their weaknesses and their strengths. The exercise which follows will be the start of learning about themselves under the umbrella of sociability.

EXERCISE 1

Party Invitations

The purpose of this exercise is to give each child the opportunity to experience what it would be like to 'be' somebody else. In the process it is interesting to observe the choice of role that the children make.

METHOD
Explain to the children it is near the end of the school term and the school have invited each child to an 'end of term' party. Ask the children to think of someone whom they would like to be in their own class, and then find a partner and consider meeting a friend at the party. The child must then role play the person they would like to be. The role play begins by each child introducing themselves but by role playing as already stated.

When you feel the children are in role ask them to say a few things about 'their real' self but staying in role. After a short verbal interchange form a circle and ask the children to state who they role played and some of their conversations.

For example Graham decided to role play Ian the classroom 'bully'. This was interesting in itself because Graham is very quiet, mumbles his speech and seeks out activities which isolate him from the other children. Graham role playing Ian went on to say how he found Graham to be a 'clever clogs', who never wanted to play games when asked, therefore suggesting he was 'too good' for the other children. When we formed a circle and the partners started to feedback conversations Graham with encouragement from the therapists started to say how difficult it was to join in games because he was frightened of doing things wrong, or being ridiculed by his peers.

CONCLUSION

From this exercise the following points are of importance.
1 The child can identify someone who they would like to be therefore acknowledging another child's strengths or weaknesses.
2 It allows the child the opportunity to gain insight into someone else's expectations of them.
3 The role play emphasises a real situation—the school party. Often this social situation is a fearful situation particularly for the likes of Graham. Practise can only increase self-confidence.
4 Working in pairs is less threatening and therefore helps to break down social barriers.
5 The sharing of information at the end encourages support from the rest of the children who are more than likely to be in a very similar position.

ROLES

Children in families are not meant to have roles. They are simply meant to be children, to be themselves. It is unfortunate, therefore, that in some families children are assigned roles or indeed take on certain attributes, whether by choice or by parental design. The 'parental child' is one such example. Here the child assumes responsibility for literally looking after the emotional welfare of the parents and the rest of the family. Thus he acts as the mediator, the soother, the calming influence, the understanding one. It is a position of great power which can be easily understood, but it also a great burden to have to be responsible for the happiness and peace of mind of other members of the family. Such a child may present to his peer group as overly mature, always understanding but also appearing to carry the rest of the world on his shoulders. The child does not seem to be able to have fun, be spontaneous or indulge in the sort of childishness that his peers are always up to.

The assignment of roles to children happens in a variety of ways. The family myth is a common phenomenon. 'Wee' Jimmy is just like his Uncle Jack. He is always getting up to mischief. He can not sit still, he will not stop talking and it does not take much for him to get into fights. 'Wee' Jimmy is at this stage barely nine months old! He grows up to be like, surprise surprise, who else but Uncle Jack of course! 'Wee' Jimmy is intolerant of other children, is always getting into scrapes and makes teacher's life a misery. Then there is the child who is the organiser. He is the one who becomes the class monitor. He may or may not be the 'class grass' as well. The 'victim' child is often the most difficult to work with. The child has a history of constantly being the one who is got at, picked upon, bullied and all of this while he remains totally blameless. The story starts with the child being perhaps the lesser wanted of the children in the family. He senses this very early and shows resentment. This will probably take the form of crying, screaming or temper tantrums. He very quickly learns that this behaviour will bring its own instant reward and so it is repeated. It does not matter that some of the attention will take the form of battering. Better some attention than none at all! There is by now further unconscious realisation that his behaviour has come to serve other important functions as well. For instance he can always scream, yell and complain about his sibs when he senses the atmosphere in the home is becoming dangerously tense and hostile. All that he is aware of is that mum and dad are not very happy with each other. Indeed they may be angry with each other. It is time to provide a distraction, a smokescreen, a camouflage to avoid matters deteriorating. So he does, and what does it matter if he gets abused for his pains as long as he has temporarily restored a ceasefire in the home. In all of this there is the constant initial recognition of his own feeling of being unwanted. Many of this child's manoeuvres both at home and at school will be designed to induce the sort of response from adults, as well as from peers, which confirm this very low opinion of himself. This is familiar territory and although it is an uncomfortable position to be in it is one that he knows and will cling to. It would take a great deal of hard work, trust and security to change that self-image.

'Role play' is a useful technique to give children the opportunity to try out other roles which are unfamiliar to them. We include here an exercise called 'Moving Story' which includes role play.

EXERCISE 2

Moving Story

The idea in this exercise as in the previous one is to provide the child with an opportunity to experience the feeling of being somebody else.

The difference in this case is that the experience is of being in one's own family or one created in fantasy.

METHOD

First of all set the scene in the room by suggesting one part of the room is the stage and the other part of the room is for the 'audience' to view the play. Give the children a theme; in this case we would suggest 'The Family'.

Each member of the group is given a number—1, 2, 3, 4 ... Take time to check everyone knows their own number. Ask numbers 1, 2, and 3 to think up a story on the theme of the family. Then numbers 1, 2, and 3 start acting out their story, whilst all the other children watch. When the performance has been running for a few minutes ask number 1 to come out and be part of the audience whilst number 4 joins in the play. Number 4 then slots into the scene. After a few more minutes number 2 is asked to come out and number 5 to go in. Continue in this way allowing the story to run on until a suitable climax is reached.

After the moving story a discussion about it would help everyone to gain some insight into their own position within their family.

When we used this exercise with a group of children the story ran from a pleasant day's family outing to chaos and despair. Jean, nine years old, the oldest of three children, and to our knowledge a child who had been given the role of 'mother and father' to her sister and brothers, clearly demonstrated to us in the moving story how she would look after everyone. When this burden became too much she then had a temper tantrum putting the attention onto herself. For a few seconds she gained some attention from the 'adults' albeit negative. As the story continued Jean became once again part of the audience. She could then sit back and look at other ways of family functioning.

In our discussion time we explored the feelings about what it felt like to play mother, father, sister and other family members. This also allows the children time to relax after, as happened with this particular group, a chaotic story.

CONCLUSIONS

1 Children find role play easy and enjoyable, when perhaps adults may not find it easy or enjoyable! By using an exercise like 'Moving Story' not only can a theme be set but some structure is given for those who find free play difficult.
2 Not all the children participate at once, therefore there is an opportunity to observe family life as seen by the other children.

3   In allowing freedom to develop within the story the children will portray incidents from real life. These become helpful for the therapists in getting to know the children.
4   When a child tries out a role in the story they are able to experience what it is like to be somebody else. This may be a worthwhile experience particularly if the therapists use it in discussion time. However, Jean who could only play herself needed her peer group as well as participation in discussion time.

INTERESTS

Football is a great leveller among boys. One is expected to show affiliation with the most successful clubs. Identifying with success is almost like being a champion oneself. In any case it is important to show an interest in sporty, manly, macho stuff. Girls do not have a common denominator like football. A preliminary interest in dolls in the preschool and early primary school years gives way to other pursuits. Music and ballet become the focus for the children of the more aspirant parents. Interest in these areas carries over into preference for groups of like minded children. Attitude formation, as one can see, starts early in life; it closes the mind to other equally constructive influences and can shape ones view of life to a narrow and restricted outlook.

Children who do not share popular interests are at risk of feeling socially isolated. The bookworm or the artistic type may become the target of ridicule. Boys and girls who do not feel competent in the gymnasium come to dread the Physical Education class. It is interesting that PE remains compulsory in the majority of schools in the land. A final remark on the subject of hobbies and pastimes concerns the sexist mode in which children are brought up to believe that male and female interests lie at opposite ends of a pole rather than along a contnuum.

In the following paragraphs an exercise is described that has proved useful in allowing group members the opportunity to share with each other their own personal and diverse interests.

EXERCISE 3

Brainstorm/Hat discussion

The aim of this exercise is to provide a framework in which free and spontaneous accounts of varying personal interests and extra-curricular activities is encouraged and the group members are invited to share their experiences or suggestions with each other. The therapist as always will join in the activity.

METHOD

The group members are asked to 'Brainstorm' on the subject of extra curricular activities. It is explained to them that a period of ten minutes will be allowed in which they must concentrate on the subject in hand and shout out any ideas that come to mind on the subject regardless of whether it is of any personal interest or not.

While this is going on, a designated member of the group writes down the various suggestions on a blackboard or on a large sheet of paper. When the ten minutes are up, the group members are asked to decide on which ideas they would like to look at more closely in the next twenty minutes that is allowed for discussion. The ideas not accommodated in the current session will be held over for a future meeting.

Alternatively if the feeling is that the group members are new to each other or are otherwise inhibited from speaking freely, a hat discussion may be suggested. Each child is asked to write down, anonymously, ideas that they would like to discuss concerning their interests or hobbies. The pieces of paper are collected and placed in a hat and each child takes it in turn to pull out a sheet of paper and read from it and the group enters into a discussion on the topic.

CONCLUSIONS

1. The group permissive atmosphere allows each member to claim an interest in a subject without fear of ridicule.
2. All ideas are individual and deserving of the group's attention.
3. A group cohesiveness develops through a process of mutual sharing and a feeling of fun and relaxation.
4. Ideas may be used as future projects for the group as a whole.

RELIGION

This can be a source of great divisiveness among children. The racism that is generated on religious grounds can spill over into life in the classroom and in the community. Children are sometimes required to assume the role of defenders of the faith. Judaism, Catholicism, Islam and some of the Christian denominations can be rigorous in the instillation of their beliefs. Clearly, there is a sense of security that derives from firmly held beliefs. However matters can be taken a step too far when children through conscious or unconscious instruction are expected to become the standard bearers of their respective religions.

In the classroom and in the community arguments over the presumed superiority of one religion over another lead to strife and segregation. In many parts of Britain today, this segregation on religious grounds is a way of life. Children attend denominational schools, make denominational friends and support denominational clubs. In Scotland, Celtic FC equals Catholic while Rangers is Protestant. In England, Arsenal FC equals Jewish while neighbouring Tottenham is Protestant.

It is difficult to say whether groupwork with children can help deal with some of the problems mentioned above. The following exercise may however be useful where progress in the group is being halted because of religious differences.

EXERCISE 4

Spectrum

The purpose of this exercise is to equate religion and religious practice with all of those other features of everyday life and personal characteristics that the individual brings to the group. The children bring in their heirarchy of values that have been given to them and hopefully go away with these values rearranged in their own mind in a way that makes them feel comfortable.

METHOD

The children are asked to consider an imaginary line extending from one end of the room to the other. This line represents a spectrum of feelings, fact or opinion. One end of the line is designated 0% and the other end is designated 100%. Various parameters are selected along which the children (and therapists) will rate themseves. Parameters dealing with religious belief and practice are accompanied with those dealing with general likes and dislikes. For example:

Church on Sunday _____ No Church on Sunday
Celtic Supporter _____ Rangers Supporter
Like Maths _____ Don't like Maths
Sunday School _____ No Sunday School
Like takeaway fish and chips ___ Don't like takeaway fish and chips

Each child is asked to place himself along the imaginary line. One parameter at a time is examined. Time is allowed for the group to observe where everybody is placed along the line. The children are asked whether they would like to change positions. When everyone is satisfied the group gathers round and a discussion follows. The exercise is repeated for each or any of the parameters chosen. The same exercise may be carried out using pen and paper for the imaginary lines although we have found that the children enjoy the physical activity of moving around the room, chatting and generally mixing with each other.

CONCLUSIONS

1 The relaxed atmosphere and the physical activity of moving around allows for disclosure of personal likes and dislikes.
2 The group members get to know things about each other that they might otherwise be hard placed to find out.
3 A sense of trust and comradeship develops in that personal issues have been disclosed and discussed without cyniscism.
4 Group members discover that there are more ways in which they are like each other than different and this often includes religious beliefs and practices. Where there are prominent differences these can be aired and discussed.

DRESS

Children are sometimes dressed according to their parents' preference. Thus a parent might wish to maintain a child as an infant through difficulties in separation and dress an eight year old boy in clothes more appropriate to a five year old. Needless to say that boy will be teased by his peers. More commonly a boy might wish to be seen as the toughie in the group and wear the necessary outfit. This appearance is often taken at face value and can serve to alienate the boy from other children and adults. The fact that the child is seeking an identity may appear to be common-sense, but the reaction he evokes from others do not always take this into account. Similarly the girl who is dressed up like a 'little doll' is not being granted any favours. As mentioned earlier the child is open to the models provided by those around her and it is not far-fetched to suggest that the 'little doll' like girl will grow up to be the 'little doll' like woman. The purpose of the following is to make the other children aware of how important appearances can be. Dress maketh the man!

EXERCISE 5

I see you

The aim in this exercise is to invite group members to comment on each others dress with a view to gaining feedback on how they present along with suggestions on how they might change if necessary. The therapists set the stage for the kind of comments that might be made.

METHOD
Prepare three cards with the following writing on them:

A It is clear that you . . .
B I discovered that you . . .
C I imagine that you . . .

Ask the children to seat themselves in a circle. Ask for one volunteer. The volunteer will be the one who has the cards read out to them. Explain that each child will have a turn to have the cards read to them. Introduce the themes physique and dress before issuing the cards. The two are complementary therefore it is not quite so obvious dress is being singled out.

Card A is then passed around the rest of the children. Each child starts off by saying 'It is clear that you' and then completes the rest of the statement. Then the B and C cards are used in the same way. It may be useful for the therapist to speak first to indicate what is required.

For example: It is clear that you wear grey trousers.
I discovered that you like to wear trousers.
I imagine that you don't like to wear school uniform.

CONCLUSIONS

1 Each child hears how others see them, which will create a picture for that child of how they must look to the others.
2 It is a shared activity with no-one being singled out and each individual is given an opportunity to speak.

3   The therapist joins in which allows every one of the group members to feel safe. The therapist provides cues which are non-threatening and so saves group members from embarrassment.
4   The cards act as a focus, again reducing intimidation.

MANNER

Often the main recollection one has of a meeting with a stranger is the demeanour that was conveyed at the time. A cheerful disposition is well remembered, as is a sulky or disgruntled one. The manner of the individual is like a calling card. It is interesting that first meetings can generate instant likes and dislikes without knowing anything at all about the individual concerned. First impressions can often last. A self-fulfilling prophetic relationship may develop along the lines of the initial feelings and reactions.

We have found in working with groups of children that, on the occasions when two children meeting for the first time experience feeings of mistrust or hostility, it has subsequently taken ages before they have been able to recognise other more likeable features about each other. Temperament does play a significant part in how the child presents to his peer group. Not all children are born leaders and not all children are self-assured. It can be extremely difficult for the shy child. It does not help to be reserved. Equally the intrusive child will be disliked. Perhaps the worst off is the infantile, demanding irritating child! By comparison the moody child comes to be recognised as such and is able to recover distance during the better spells. What is important to note is that, given temperament as well as the family background and upbringing, the child is nevertheless open to the influence of both his peers and the other adults who have the care of him for the time that he is away from home.

A drawing exercise will help to explore the attitude of how a child is seen by others. By looking at this area it is hoped that a child will gain strength from the feedback and therefore be able to adapt himself in order to create more positive and warm feelings towards himself especially on first meetings when that first impression lingers on.

EXERCISE 6

Who's Who

The idea of this exercise in its use of pen and paper is to allow the children to portray graphically their perceptions of each other, with a view to each recipient benefiting from the thoughts of the others.

A Football 1.	Tennis 2.
3.	4.

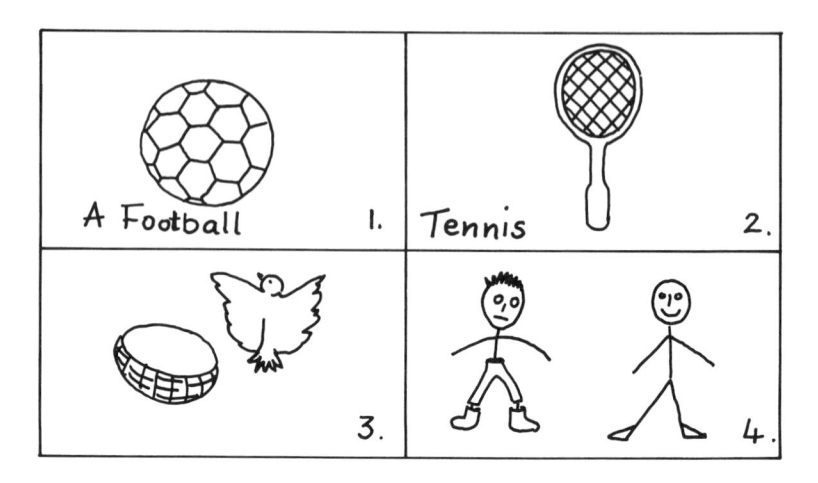

METHOD

Each person sits in a circle with a large sheet of paper in front of them. Felt tipped pens should be freely available. Each person puts their own name on the top of the paper. The paper is then moved to the next person on their left.

What the group then sees is a paper with someone else's name at the top. Now it is time to think about the person of that name and draw a picture of how they present to the individual. The drawings may be concrete or symbolic, but tell the children they will explain to each other the meaning behind their drawings. Keep passing the pictures to the left until each person has a paper in front of them with their own name on and a number of drawings.

The next stage is to explore the meanings behind the drawings.

We have found the drawing side of the exercise to be easy once everyone understands the concept. However, help is often needed to put the pictures into words, and from the words extract a meaning. The therapist will have to be aware of this and tease out positive explanations. It is important to look at each drawing and receive explanations, because drawings are not always flattering!

The four drawings represent Paul, a ten year old boy who originally

SOCIETY INVITES YOU TO JOIN ITS RANKS

came to the group with a 'tough guy' image. You can see from each section that various descriptions were given about Paul:

> Section 1 illustrates how Paul had made friends with another group member by his keenness in football.
> In section 2, a tennis bat was drawn to show how Paul was considered to be a child who liked physical activity.
> Section 3, was the therapist's view of how Paul had been able to make a positive change in his life and was ready to 'leave the nest'.
> In section 4, the 'tough guy' image has gone, leaving behind a more approachable, sensitive boy.

It is important for the child to have feedback from his peers and from his carers on how he comes across to other people; on the impressions that he creates, good or bad, and how he might improve. The narcissistic position has got to be challenged. The child who is made to feel omnipotent enjoys his power but also suffers by it.

CONCLUSIONS

1. Each child is given the opportunity to think about someone else, then put their thoughts onto paper and at a later stage verbalise those thoughts.
2. The therapist is also given an opportunity to feedback some information about the children.
3. It allows a chance to release feelings about another which may have been repressed, therefore bringing about change in the way one deals with someone.
4. Often drawing is an activity which is less threatening than just talking, especially to the quiet child who does not like to speak out.

ADDITIONAL EXERCISES

Polio

This exercise was brought to the group by the children as a game that is often seen in the playground.

METHOD

One child volunteers to stand at the far end of the room while the others wait in a group at the other end. The child at the far end shouts out a topic, for example, cars, and the rest of the group choose various makes of car, e.g. Ford, Mini, Porsche, etc. When all have chosen, the list is shouted out to the child at the far end who may decide to choose one of the makes of car for himself. For example, should he choose the Mini, then the child already identified as the mini races to change places with the child at the far end. Whoever reaches the respective place first wins and is then in a position to repeat the whole process again with a fresh topic!

As one can imagine, there is considerable interaction between the children in this game. The main body of children have to work together, while everybody gets a chance to direct the group in terms of choosing a topic. The game is also quite exhausting and enjoyable.

Coming as it does from the playground, this game has an inbuilt code that enhances the socialisation process. It can also be suitably modified to help deal with problems relating to Sociability, Interests, Roles and Manner.

Hugee Bear

METHOD

One child volunteers to be Hugee Bear. Depending on the subject in hand, Hugee Bear is asked to shout out something like, for instance, to do with dress, so that he says, HUGEE BEAR: WHITE SOCKS. All the children with white socks hug each other. Another item of clothing is selected and the process is repeated

The Hugee Bear topics could centre around themes to do with dress, religious interests and sociability. The Therapist could encourage and direct the group to choose relevant topics.

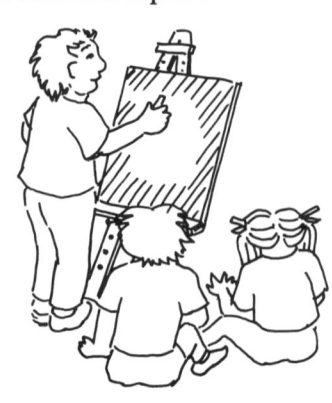

6 The trauma of *loss*

The concept of loss is much more widely understood now than it was, say, even a decade ago. No doubt this has been due to work done on bereavement in terms of the research into its effects on the family, the increasing use of bereavement counselling and most importantly perhaps the conveying of the message which says that society must allow for its members openly to experience the grief that comes from such loss and that this experience is publicly and socially acceptable. The question that arises is whether the same can be said for all the other kinds of losses that occur as part and parcel of everyday life. Loss through separation and divorce, from moving house or losing a pet, from changing school and losing friends, from temporary or permanent separations from the family for whatever reasons, from changing foster homes, children's home, residential schools or even from repeated hospitalisation. The list is endless and the main question for the purposes of this chapter is, to what extent is the nature of loss and the problems that can stem from it, understood as it applies to children and their personality and emotional development?

In this section we shall be looking at some of the problems associated with loss through parental separations, through divorce, from death of a family member and also from miscellaneous situations that while remaining unexplored can have traumatic consequences.

PARENTAL SEPARATION

It may be said that in the short term at least, the uncertainty associated with parental separation is more difficult for the child to cope with than the finality of a divorce, or the reality of death. Often in cases of parental separation there will have been previous rows, arguments, threats of and actual 'trial' separations with attempts at (some successful) reconciliations. The child in the family will have experienced a repeating cycle of emotions ranging from guilt at feeling responsible for parental dissatisfaction with each other, to sadness at feeling the family hurt, to anger and then despair at feeling rejected and deserted by the leaving parent. Much of this emotional experience will be reflected in the child's behaviour at school in relation to significant adults, i.e., teachers, who could become equated with parents, to peers equated with sibs, to school performance in assuming a couldn't care less attitude. The problem of understanding the child's behaviour at this stage, however, is complicated by the fact that he is likely to keep secret this aspect of his life in fear of the stigma that is associated with such situations but more so in the hope that given time, all may come right in the end.

The following exercise is aimed at helping the child begin to acknowledge the home situation and the implications behind the parents' separation. This exercise could also be used to look at the effects of divorce.

Family Sculpture—Using Chairs

With the children seated in a circle explain to the children that they are going to spend some time sculpting their family with chairs. At this point it will be necessary to clarify the word 'sculpture' by giving examples such as placing out as many chairs as will represent the size of the child's family; placing the chairs out in relation to how close each member of the family is; placing out the chairs to demonstrate how the family get on together; if the chairs are coloured perhaps different colours, could represent moods (red—angry, yellow—happy, blue—sad); if the chairs are different size perhaps the size of chair may be able to represent something to the child. There are many variables and you will find once the children get started, their own ideas will emerge. Allow at least fifteen minutes for each child to have a turn if they feel capable of doing so.

Start by asking for a volunteer. There is usually one volunteer in a group who will set the ball rolling. Ask the rest of the children to sit at the back of the room to allow space for the sculpt. The leader should stand near to the child to give non-verbal encouragement and to clarify any feelings the child may have. Once the sculpt is complete go around with the child asking him to clarify and tell the group who the chairs belong to.

When the sculpt is complete encourage group questions about the sculpted family set up. Obviously the leader will aim to bring out specific difficulties the child may be experiencing, such as parental separation. The rest of the children may find question time valuable to help them clarify their own family difficulties.

The last child to volunteer is usually the one who finds this technique

THE TRAUMA OF *LOSS* 55

threatening. However, if you ask the group if they would like that child to do a family sculpt and all the children agree, you will find the child perhaps with some reluctance getting up and doing it. From experience this is the child who keeps the family situation a secret in the hope things will improve. End the session by sitting back in a circle and asking if anyone wants to say anything else about families.

Tim

Tim fits into the category of the child who is last to volunteer and has recently had to face parental upset, resulting in separation. He has also been quiet at home. When it comes to Tim's turn about discussions he is persuaded by the group to have a go. Tim sets out his family as follows:

    x Mum   x Tim   x Mum's brother   x Dad
              x Hamster

Tim was obviously quite angry that Dad had gone away. Interestingly, he had adopted Mum's unmarried brother for some male support and identity. At question time Julie, who had already said that her Dad had gone away, was the first to ask Tim about why Dad was far away from the family group. Tim in his reply was able to release his feelings about Dad, whilst at the same time clarify for Julie that she wasn't the only one to experience family disharmony.

CONCLUSIONS

1. By sculpting the family, the child is able to clarify for himself how he feels and fits into the family situation.
2. The leader is able to offer support and act as a facilitator to encourage discussions of family dynamics.
3. Allowing each child to take a turn at sculpting and sharing their families with others, encourages communication and group cohesiveness.
4. Sharing gives the child the opportunity to realise that others may have had similar experiences. This makes the situation less of a social stigma.

DIVORCE

The loss of a parent through divorce can result in problems that are emotional, developmental, social and financial. The last two aspects mentioned could easily be overlooked. Society has yet to make adequate provision for the single-parent family and perhaps this slowness to do so reflects the basic difficulty of society in accepting the notion of the split family. As mentioned previously, this difficulty is then reflected in the stigma of belonging to such a family. At a more concrete level, the financial loss arising parents divorcing brings in its wake its own train of events, from the major business of moving house to the lesser but equally important problems of restricted finances for food, clothing, toys and pocket-money. At the developmental level, the absence of the same sexed parent can, for example, in boys give rise to the need to strive for excessive masculinity. The lack of the opposite sexed parent will, though some may dispute this, deprive the child of the opportunity of modelling and identification that will be important in the making of satisfactory, future heterosexual relationships and the establishing of a happy family life. Emotionally speaking the child of the divorced couple will have experienced all the feelings mentioned previously in the run up to the divorce. It is important to work through these feelings if the child is not to be left in a position of anger, distrust and low self-esteem. One of the problems associated with divorcing couples is that of the custody battles that sometimes rage on, causing uncertainty, confusion and split loyalties for the child. A recent development in this connection is the 'Conciliation' Service that is meant to help resolve some of these problems.

The aim of this exercise is to help the child put his new family situation into perspective and allow the opportunity to express feelings about the divorce.

Symbolic Family Drawings

When the children are seated in a circle ask the children to close their eyes and think about their own family members. They are to think what each member reminds them of, other than real people. A few examples may help their thought processes, e.g., perhaps someone who has left home may be a butterfly; perhaps a baby may feature as a football rattle; perhaps someone the child does not want to leave will be a piece of elastic. The first thing that comes to mind is the one to put down on paper. There should be various art materials for the task to allow freedom of expression. The drawing continues until all family members are on paper.

Some examples of children's symbolic families:

Simon aged 10

Dad — spanner
likes cars

Simon — clown
likes to tell jokes

(younger) brother — toys (cars)
likes playing with cars

Mum — cooking pot
likes to spend all her time in the kitchen

Gran — wool
always knitting jumpers

The next stage is for each child to share his symbolic family with the group. The leader who will do the exercise with the children could provide a model for the children by talking about their own symbolic family first. Questions from other group members should be invited alongside those of leader. The purpose is to tease out feelings about divorce.

CONCLUSIONS

1 By using symbols the child views the exercise as fun and the threatening element of exposing oneself is reduced.
2 It is often easier to talk about objects rather than people and, therefore, the symbols give permission to open out and explore feelings.
3 By sharing the family scene, children are able to see that there are different styles of families with some aspects that have similarities to their own.

DEATH OF A FAMILY MEMBER

The child's reaction to the death of a family member will to some extent depend on his age and stage of cognitive development. Some people may argue that children do not understand the concept of death before reaching the age of six to eight years. What is certainly clear, however, is that the experience and feeling of loss is a reality even for a new-born infant when it becomes aware of the temporary absence of its significant care taking figure.

The death of a family member, particularly in the nuclear family, will precipitate the common feelings of grief and sadness, anger and guilt, and the eventual resolution of these feelings in all the family members. This, broadly speaking, could be regarded as a healthy outcome and indeed entails a lot of hard work. In the event of a parental death, for instance, the surviving parent has to cope with personal grief as well as that experienced by the children. Help and support in this task may or may not be forthcoming. Priorities may get confused so that personal loss may come before the child's loss and vice versa. Relationships with the deceased member may have been ambivalent with one or more surviving members of the family which would complicate the grieving process further. The child may be used to parent the adult or alternatively to attribute with sad and/or resentful feelings well beyond the point at which that child has successfully adjusted to the immediate crisis.

These and other obstacles to the normal grieving process will be reflected in the child's behaviour in a variety of ways—sadness, tearfulness and misery within and outwith the home, psychosomatic disturbance necessitating repeated visits to the GP, school refusal, poor academic performance, behavioural problems at school and at home.

EXERCISE

Death for some children is easily mentioned within a group, although there are children who remain silent when the subject is raised. However, once the topic of death is opened up most children have had someone die or a pet die and, therefore, have material for group sharing. The following exercise is used to help explore death, in the context of other life events.

'Life Map'

When the group are seated in a circle ask them to decide upon symbols to represent life events. Using birth as an example, encourage the group to agree on a drawing to illustrate birth. Someone draws the picture and from then on the children are encouraged to think of other happenings. Considering death, the leader may say, 'I remember when my dog died; has anyone else had a similar experience?' When the life events drawings are finished, the children take pens and paper to make a map of their own life events.

After each map is completed discussion is encouraged. In this instance, death is the important issue, therefore, the leader will help the group to focus more on this topic.

CONCLUSIONS

1 Discussing death openly in a group takes away the idea of it being a taboo subject.
2 Most children have at some stage experienced a death and to be able to share it with their own peer group allows their own ideas to emerge, rather than be tangled up in their parents' attitude towards death.
3 The first part of the exercise warms the children up to being more relaxed to explore emotive issues.

60 CHILDREN NEED GROUPS

Examples of children's symbols for 'life map'.

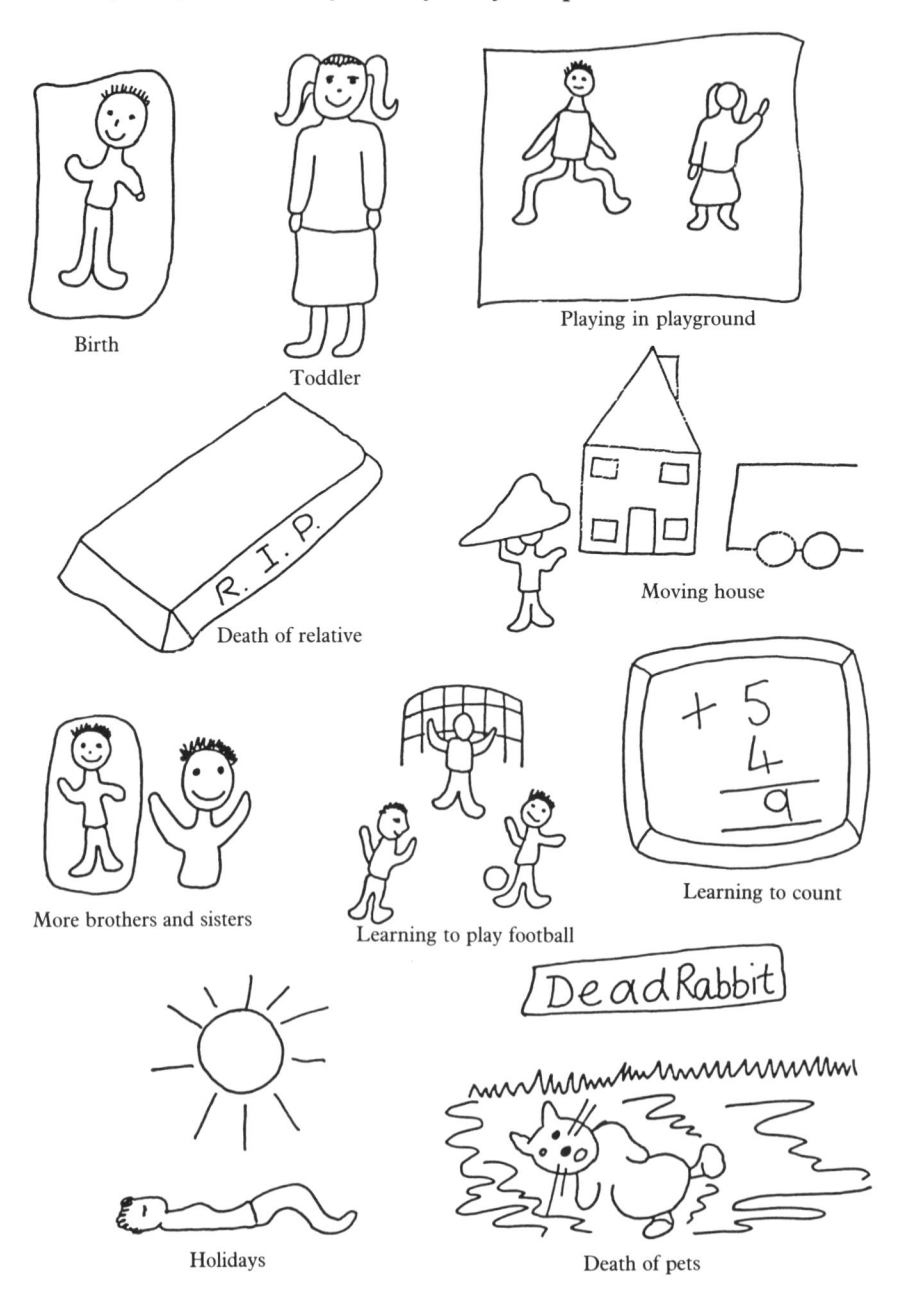

Birth

Toddler

Playing in playground

Death of relative

Moving house

More brothers and sisters

Learning to play football

Learning to count

Holidays

Death of pets

4   Being able to identify with another child who has lost someone close will bring further comfort to the child.

MISCELLANEOUS LOSS

Under this heading a common form of loss encountered is that involved in moving house. The stress for the child and his family is two-fold. Firstly, there is the coming to terms with giving up the familiarity and security of the old home, and its neighbourhood, separating from friends, leaving the old school and all that goes with it. What follows and is probably the most difficult is the process of adjustment to the new situation. Whereas some children might regard the whole process as a great adventure, there are others who would fear the prospect of the new challenge. There is much to be said for maintaining the sameness of the environment for some children and where this is disturbed by moves of home, school performance may suffer and behavioural problems occur. Helping to adjust remains essentially a family task but in some cases outside agencies may be asked to help.

Among the less common forms of loss, two categories are mentioned but not enlarged upon as these are specialist subjects that are covered in the relevant books. The first is the whole area of children in Care, in children's homes or in foster homes, where there has been an ultimate breakdown in the relationship between child and family and where the loss is incurred by the child and his family and the cost must be met albeit with help from the appropriate agencies. The second category is that of the chronic and continuous loss suffered by children with emotional and material deprivation, much of this occurring in private and out of the public eye. It is fortunate, therefore, that the different professions and the courts are now actively co-ordinating their efforts to identify and help these children and their families.

The following exercise can be adapted to fit miscellaneous situations.

'The Auction'

The leader writes down a list of headings relative to the group and blue-tacks them on a large sheet of paper. The headings may be as follows:

New school	New home	New friends
Old school	Old home	Old friends
Happiness	Dad	Mum
Grandparents	Brother	Sister
Family Together	Own toys	

62 CHILDREN NEED GROUPS

These are obviously a group of emotive topics and, therefore, some lighter topics may be included such as:

| Holiday | Seeing a film | Staying up later |
| More pocket money | New bike | A puppy, etc. |

When the list is complete, it should be placed in front of the group for them to ponder over. The leader gives each person fifty tokens with which to acquire anything on the list they would value. The leader starts the bidding off. When a heading is won it is taken off the sheet and given to the child. The appropriate points are given in payment. The child can bid for as many things as he would like, but when their points run out they have to stop bidding.

The auction is complete when no-one has any points left. The children are then asked to sit in a circle and share with the rest of the group what they obtained and the reasons why they wanted it. The group should be allowed to ask each other questions, whilst the leader helps to encourage discussion at an emotional level.

CONCLUSIONS

1 The exercise can be made to suit the individual needs within the group.
2 From experience, the first part of the exercise is usually fun to do. Therefore the group are well warmed-up to start thinking more about why they want certain things.
3 The exercise clarifies for the child the situation of loss, be it school, parent, friends and, therefore, allowing a release of feelings.
4 The responsibility placed on the child to obtain what he wants makes the item seem more precious and, therefore, helps to develop feelings of awareness.
5 The exercise encourages assertiveness and decision-making.

ADDITIONAL EXERCISES

For the younger child the use of the following nursery-rhyme may help facilitate an understanding of the concept of loss and the discussion that follows could gently bring home the reality of that loss.

Humpty-Dumpty

Encourage the children to be actively involved in singing this rhyme.

> Humpty-Dumpty sat on a wall
> Humpty-Dumpty had a great fall.
> All the King's horses and all the King's men,
> Couldn't put Humpty together again.

All the children could hold hands and move around in a circle. When the verse is said (a number of times to stimulate the children) a group discussion would follow about what has happened to Humpty-Dumpty and, in particular, relating this to everyday life such as the loss of a family member.

CONCLUSIONS

1. The Nursery-rhyme is familiar and children will find it easy to relate to.
2. By using Humpty-Dumpty to explain loss, it does not directly relate to any child in particular so there is less need to become defensive.
3. It is a shared activity, encouraging communication and sharing.
4. The physical movement and verbalisation will help to reduce excess energy before the discussion about Humpty-Dumpty. This will lead to a more relaxed session.

The following exercises again for the younger child could be used to look at loss of family members through separation or death.

The Clay Family

The children are seated around a table with a suitable amount of clay for modelling. 'Play-doh' could be used as an alternative and it may be more appropriate for the younger child. Each child is requested to think about their family doing something. This may range from watching television, going to the park or on holiday. The essential part is to include all the family members. It is often easier for the child to lay the figures down on a sheet of paper and make a picture. Once the figures are completed, encourage the group to discuss their families. Relevant questions can be drawn from their pictures such as who is closest to who? where is daddy? and so on.

CONCLUSIONS

1 Clay or 'play-doh' is tactile and children usually enjoy working with this medium, and their hands. Because of this, it becomes a non-threatening and enjoyable activity.
2 By asking the picture to portray the family doing something, it will make it easier for the child to relate to.
3 At the end of the modelling each child is given the opportunity to express their feelings behind their pictures and consequently they can be encouraged to release feelings they may have regarding separation.
4 The children share their experience with each other and, therefore, have the opportunity to identify with other group members in similar situations.

Eric

Eric had recently started nursery school and just as he had begun to accept this new situation a fire occurred at home. The home was destroyed and Eric's baby brother died. After this incident, a change was seen in Eric. He became hyperactive with poor concentration and when the house was refurbished he was afraid of it. His mother was young and inexperienced, she found it difficult to cope with the loss of her baby and this led to an inability to deal with Eric's loss as well as her own. Eventually, the following idea was suggested to help both the mother and the nursery staff to deal with Eric's feelings. After a discussion with the nursery teacher and the mother, it was decided that Eric should be placed with a small group of children (two or three) with a similar religious background. The focus of the activity was for the teacher to paint a picture of heaven and for the children to say what she should include.

This activity helped Eric with the transition of thinking that his brother was still in the burnt house to going to heaven. The other children in the group, with their concrete ideas about death, made him feel more secure. By involving the mother it encouraged her to help her son, acknowledging her problem and providing some comfort for him.

7 Hospitals can be quite nice places really

In the past three or four decades, much has been written about the effects of hospitalisation on children. The general concensus of opinion is that hospitalisation can be a traumatic experience with short to long term consequences if insufficient account is taken of the child's social, cognitive and emotional needs during that child's stay in hospital. Equally it has been shown that the child can benefit from various positive aspects within the therapeutic environment, and indeed many admissions to hospital are made on the basis of respite care for children and families in difficult circumstances.

Most paediatric hospitals in Britain today are geared to providing a therapeutic environment for the child that will make their experience in hospital as least traumatic as possible. These developments have been based on discussions between paediatricians, psychologists, psychiatrists and other health workers. Thus features such as extended visiting times, accommodating the parents of the younger child, key nurse roles, educational and preparatory booklets for children due to come into hospital, playgroups and playleaders, toys, own clothes, cheerful ward decor, etc, are commonplace in most hospitals. Developments continue to take place in terms of research programmes that are encouraged to look at the effects of hospitalisation in general terms as well as more specifically in terms of its effects on the well-being of different groups of children suffering from various chronic physical illnesses.

In this chapter we shall be looking at the problems that arise during the period of hospitalisation and we shall go on to consider how structured group activities might be used to help the child cope with this experience. It may be useful, however, in the first instance, to place the experience of hospitalisation into some kind of perspective in terms of the common causes that necessitate a child's admission to hospital and which also, to a large extent, dictate the duration of that child's stay in hospital.

The child may be admitted with an acute respiratory illness of viral or bacterial origin, in respiratory distress, such as in the case of a severe asthmatic attack, or for treatment of allergies and acute allergic reactions that are common enough causes for admission. The child may be admitted for investigations of vague abdominal pains, or for investigations of pyrexia of unknown cause. On average these conditions may require the child to stay in hospital for a period of a week, barring complications. In other instances, the child may be admitted following an accident and the duration of stay in hospital will be determined by the extent of the injuries. Planned admissions may take place for corrective surgery, for orthopaedic procedures, or for dental procedures in a wide variety of conditions such as cerebral palsy, mental handicap or congenital anomalies. The child may be admitted for investigation of suspected epilepsy, for stabilising blood sugar levels and getting the right doses of drugs for conditions such as diabetes and other metabolic and endocrine problems. The child may require repeated hospitalisation for illnesses resulting in such conditions as cystic fibrosis, renal problems, leukaemia and so on. These children may well require much longer periods of stay in hospital.

It is clear then from the above that there are certain conditions that come on suddenly and that require hospitalisation for brief periods of time whereas there are other illnesses which are rather more chronic and require not only repeated hospitalisation but require the child to stay in hospital for considerable lengths of time. Also it is clear that the nature of the illness, the degree of stress and the type of investigative procedures such as blood taking to lumbar punctures will determine the degree of trauma that the child experiences. All of these factors must be taken into account when considering the experience of the child's stay in hospital, given that for obvious reasons each child's experience will be uniquely personal.

Let us now go on to consider some of the more common problems encountered during the child's stay in hospital, in general terms such as separation difficulties, regression, behavioural problems and more specifically problems relating to surgery, medical investigative and treatment procedures, and the group of children who remain chronically disabled or who have chronic physical illnesses.

SEPARATION DIFFICULTIES

This kind of difficulty is usually encountered with the pre-school child. The younger the child the more vulnerable he is to separation from significant caretaker figures and from familiar surroundings. The management problems result from separation difficulties present in the form of distress experienced, and manifested by the child at various stages of the hospitalisation process, for example, being separated from mother at the close of visiting times, or the distress experienced during medical procedures which may well be perceived by the child as a physical attack on its body. It is by now well known that the young child goes through the three phases of protest, despair and denial upon being separated from its parents while in hospital. In the first stage the child cries loudly or has tantrums in 'protest', while in the second stage the child may well have given up in 'despair', feeling either abandoned or that the parent is unlikely to return, while in the third phase the internal distress is so great that the child can cope with this only by 'denial', so that he or she is likely to appear to have recovered from the previous two stages and is now behaving with apparent normality.

Normally the child's experience of separation difficulties will be influenced by factors already mentioned in the above paragraphs, namely the nature of the illness, the duration of stay and the procedures involved. Additional and probably crucial factors are the relationship that existed prior to hospitalisation between the child and its family and the significant caretaking figure. In the event of this relationship having been fragile, it is likely that the experience of hospitalisation will only serve to make the world appear an even more hostile and rejecting place for the child. In many hospitals now it is acceptable practice for one or both parents to be able to stay in the hospital with the young child to offset separation difficulties. This may not always be possible, however, for the parents who have to look after their other young children in the home. It is important, therefore, that the role of the key nurse assigned to look after the child is an appropriate substitute figure, providing the child with a stable and nurturing relationship that may help offset some of the child's feelings of being abandoned. For the child of four or five years of age it is possible to introduce a group activity to distract and help the child understand and cope with the experience of being separated from his family.

Painting a picture of your home

Sitting the small group of children around a table or together on the floor, the therapist begins by saying to the children that we are going to paint a picture of your house and your family, stressing the importance of the family situation. The children should be allowed a free range of painting materials to allow freedom of expression. When painting the pictures with young children the child's representation of a scene will often be difficult to perceive. Therefore care and sensitivity must be taken when discussing the pictures.

Once the pictures are finished the therapist asks each child to say something about their home and family. If there are children in the group who find talking difficult identity the most vocal child and ask them to talk first. Another way to encourage verbalisation would be for the therapist to describe their own picture therefore presenting the children with a model. The therapist goes on to encourage the children to ask questions about the other children's pictures, thereby bringing more feelings of home life to the surface.

Donald

Five year old Donald had had many hospital admissions within his short life. His latest admission had been for treatment of a serious illness. While Donald was now physically much better and he was out of danger, Donald's mother felt distressed by his behaviour. Whenever she went away Donald became clingy and weepy. On her return he would ignore her or become aggressive towards her.

Donald had been encouraged to join the painting group and paint his home and family. During the painting he was quiet and thoroughly absorbed with the task. However, when it was time to share the pictures Donald only managed to say, 'I'm not going home', and masses of tears followed the statement. The therapist was able to reassure Donald that he would go home and one little girl in the group said, 'We only stay here for a few days'. This experience was important for Donald in that he allowed his repressed feelings to surface. When his mother returned Donald and mother began talking which was a relief for both of them.

CONCLUSIONS

1 Painting a picture of home and the family reinforces the idea that hospital admission is not permanent.
2 The picture becomes the focus and therefore less threatening. Young children find it easier to talk about a painting than talk about how they feel.

3 By sharing the same experience the children are made to feel that they are not alone with their anxieties.
4 The pictures could be put up in a corner and could be referred to, providing a constant reminder of home and further reinforcement.
5 Feedback from the child could help the parents and other hospital staff gain a greater understanding of the child's inner world.

REGRESSION

Hospitals are of necessity regimented places and have routines with which most of us are unfamiliar, but with which we have to comply. The most difficult aspect perhaps of being in hospital is the loss of independence, the giving up of control and the placing of oneself in the charge of others. For the adult who has developed a self-concept and who understands the temporary nature of the situation, these problems may be something that he or she can cope with. For the child, however, who has yet to develop a proper concept of time and of personal identity, the hospitalisation period seems both interminable as well as threatening in its attack on the child's sense of autonomy and independent functioning.

Regression can manifest in a variety of ways, although the phenomenon itself seems to stem from feelings of dependency, and loss of control that are fostered in the highly routined environment of hospitals. Thus many hospitals in recognising this problem, have developed a more flexible routine so that children are able to, for instance, wear their own clothes, bring in their own toys, have flexible sleeping and eating arrangements and are encouraged to follow their tailor-made educational programmes where applicable so that they do not fall too far behind when they return to school.

If regression can be regarded as arising from a crises of competence then the symptoms may reflect a state of helplessness in which the child gives up responsibility for himself in favour of being completely looked after. This may include behaving in a way which is not appropriate to age, having disregard for appearance and hygiene, developing food fads, developing toileting problems and falling behind educationally, etc. When these symptoms emerge it is important to provide the child with the kind of experience in which he is reassured of his own feeling of competence. This may take the form of group exercises in which the child, along with others, is given the opportunity to demonstrate confidence in himself and his abilities.

The aim of the next exercise is to find a way of working out alternative and more effective ways of dealing with hospitalisation. As previously stated, social skills have a tendency to disappear and a child becomes dependent on adults for daily chores.

'Make believe play'

Set aside a child size domestic corner in the hospital playroom and equip it with cooking items, items related to cleaning self and toileting facilities. The therapist will set the scene by suggesting to the children it would be a good idea to play mummies, daddies and children at home. Allow the children to choose their parts and allow play to develop spontaneously. The therapist may think it appropriate to encourage the children to change roles. The play should be wound down when the children start to show signs of restlessness. It would be important to share the play with the children at the end by suggesting sitting, talking and sharing.

The older child would feel that this type of play is 'babyish' therefore the following exercise may be useful for them.

'Hospital likes and dislikes'

The children are invited to sit around a table. Each child is given a pencil and paper. The paper is divided into two. One side of the paper is headed 'likes' and the other is headed 'dislikes'. Each child is asked to write down five things they like most about being in hospital and five things they dislike most. The information is then used for discussion. Perhaps a play could develop from the theme of 'likes and dislikes'.

Some examples of hospital likes and dislikes

Five likes
1 playing pool
2 going to occupational therapy
3 computer
4 picnics
5 the nurses

Five dislikes
1 beds
2 school
3 food
4 get up too early
5 drugs

Five more Likes
1 the picnic
2 the lunches
3 playing games
4 visitors
5 the nurses

Five more Dislikes
1 cold food
2 too hot
3 noisy babies
4 being inside
5 miss my goldfish

CONCLUSIONS—BOTH EXERCISES

1   There is opportunity for communication. Verbal expression of feelings is encouraged without it being threatening.
2   An opportunity to release feelings, either through role play or by writing them down.
3   to encourage self-awareness of one's own situation and to gain awareness of the other children's position.
4   The play/writing elements are stimulating activities and create an opportunity to be less preoccupied with oneself.
5   The re-enactment for the pre-school child of familiar domestic routines and the opportunity presented to the older child to assert his feelings about hospital life, within the confines of the group, allows the children a recognition of their feeling state, as well as the opportunity to recover a measure of control over their own lives.

BEHAVIOURAL PROBLEMS

These problems can fall into two main categories; namely those precipitated by the change of environment with new rules and regulations, following the child's admission to hospital, and those problems that the child brings with him to the hospital which will have been manifested elsewhere, e.g. at home and at school. The first category will also be a reflection of the child's difficulties in separating from his family as well as a result of regressing due to a feeling of loss of control and autonomy. Thus the problems encountered will be among those already mentioned, such as non-compliance with medication and with other hospital routines such as going to bed at the appropriate time, having a balanced diet, etc. There may also be resistance to treatment and investigative procedures, shows of aggression to other children or staff, or alternatively withdrawn or solitary behaviour in terms of not socialising with the rest of the ward population. It is important that these problems be understood in the context in which they arise and group exercises have already been suggested to help the children cope with these difficulties.

Problem behaviours that the child brings with him will usually have already been a cause for concern in the child's home environment and at school. These problems, however, seem magnified in the hospital setting where there are other children to be cared for who are ill and in need of attention. The etiology of these problems has to be found in family and other circumstances and are referred to in appropriate chapters of this book. The problems complained of usually fall within the categories of conduct and neurotic disorders like non co-operative or aggressive behaviour teasing and bullying, fearful, withdrawn and solitary behaviour. Clearly it is difficult to 'treat' the child for these behaviours while he is in hospital for other, physical, reasons but it may be useful to have some group exercises that will help the child to become aware of and to learn to modify his behaviour within the hospital environment.

1 THE PRE-SCHOOL CHILD

The aim of the exercise is to bring together a small group of children to perform a shared task and encourage positive behaviour. During this stage children are ready to be involved with their peers and begin to understand sharing.

The task—a 3D picture

The therapist asks the children to sit in a circle round a large sheet of paper. The children are given age appropriate materials such as building blocks, toy people, toy animals and paints which could be used for a background colour. The therapist asks the group to complete the task on the paper using the materials provided. The task may be to build a hospital or a street of houses, or a trip to the seaside. The task should have a group theme. One would expect ideas for the theme to be generated by the children, but this may have to be teased out of them by the therapist. Themes could be linked to the home situation, life in hospital or outings with the family. Children within the group should be allowed to have their own ideas but the sharing element must be emphasised. A place in the room should be set aside to display the work. Parents should be encouraged to share the completed task with their child.

2 THE SCHOOL-AGE CHILD

Here the child's skills are becoming more sophisticated and the child plays spontaneously with other children. The idea of belonging and working within a group is more acceptable and general behaviour is more sensible and independent.

The task—a group collage

Ask the children to join together in a circle with a large sheet of paper placed in the centre of the circle. Again the theme for the collage will be teased out of the children by the therapist. Similar themes as previously disccused could be encouraged. Fantasy themes may develop and these could be usefully encouraged as a group theme. One would expect more sharing to develop alongside the demonstrating of own skills. For the collage a varied range of materials could be used such as dried footstuffs, use of scissors, magazines to cut up and so on.

CONCLUSIONS

1 The children are allowed to demonstrate skills. Therefore, they will feel more competent and experience their own strengths.
2 Interacting with their peers will continue the social learning process, and encourage more positive behaviour.
3 Being an autonomous group without nursing or medical interference will encourage development of competence.
4 The tasks are aimed at the children's developmental level. Therefore, they are familiar, feel safe and not threatening.
5 Depending on the collage created, a variety of feelings may be expressed regarding separation, loss, disappointment, frustrations, etc. These feelings can be discussed and linked to behaviours that occur on the ward with suggestions from the group on how best to cope with such feelings in more constructive and appropriate ways.

SURGERY

The term surgery has connotations for invasiveness and attack, albeit representing a procedure that is a necessary part of the healing process. The fact that most surgery will be carried out under general anaesthetic, is another cause for concern and exaggerates the child's fantasies about what is being done to him while he is asleep and out of control. These problems are further complicated by the pain and discomfort that accompanies such a process. The whole business begins to sound and feel punitive and questions begin to arise in the child's mind about whether he has done something wrong to deserve this punishment. Nightmares are a common enough occurrence in children who have had or are about to undergo surgery. The period of adjustment, physical and psychological, following surgery can be short or long depending on various factors. One important factor is the amount of preparation that the child receives prior to being admitted to hospital, especially in the case of planned admissions where the parents have the opportunity to prepare the child for the hospitalisation process. This process can be further helped by nursing and medical staff conveying both to the parents and to the child in simple and readily understandable but non-threatening ways, the nature of the condition the child is suffering from, the reasons why surgery is indicated and a summary of how the procedure will be carried out to effect a cure of the condition.

'Exploring your body'

Each child is given a large sheet of paper big enough to lie on and draw around their body. Discarded wallpaper rolls can be useful for this exercise.

Ask each child to find a partner and, in turn, each child draws round the other child. Thus producing a life size body image. When all the children have their own body image in front of them, the next part of the exercise begins.

Ask each child to draw in all their body features and when this is completed the therapist can look at the various reasons for the children being in hospital. Working as a group but focusing on each child individually, discuss the reasons the child is in hospital and encourage the child to draw on his/her body image what is likely to happen to the particular part in the surgical process. While allowing the child to fantasise it is important for the therapist to be familiar with the case in hand so as to guide the child on the realities of the situation where necessary. At the end of the group the drawings can hang near to the child's own personal area of the ward.

CONCLUSIONS

1. The child begins to have some understanding of his/her body and how the surgical procedure is going to effect it.
2. A discussion of the procedure prior to the event, allows the children an opportunity to express their fears and fantasies and so helps relieve some of the anxieties about the actual event.
3. The completed picture by the bedside allows for discussion between child and family, resulting in a mutual kind of reassurance.

4 Post operatively, the body picture can be referred to as a check for accuracy of perceptions before and after surgery.
5 The external representation of the 'whole body' reinforces the idea of body integration with emphasis on the part of the body that is being treated while the rest of the body remains intact.

MEDICAL PROCEDURES

Medical investigative and treatment procedures firstly, can be strange, secondly, can be threatening and thirdly, they can be painful. Taking blood, giving injections, having sophisticated X-ray work, taking tablets, having drips set up, having catheters, suppositories and endoscopes, or having brain scans and EEGs are but a few of the procedures that may be involved in the child's admission to hospital. The initial medical examination can be traumatic enough in itself with the child stripped and 'exposed' as it were while the doctor palpates and manipulates various parts of the body to check that they are in working order. If these procedures are regarded as generally being one-off affairs then there are others that are painful procedures, that need to be repeated at regular intervals for the investigation or treatment of a particular condition.

Clearly it is difficult to familiarise the child, well in advance, with all the procedures that are to be used although much can and is achieved by the sympathetic and considerate handling of the child, by medical and nursing staff, at the time that the procedure is being used. One way, of course, is for the child to become familiar with representative toy equipment and the use of group games to rehearse what is likely to happen in a non-threatening environment, so that the event itself becomes less traumatic than it might otherwise have been.

'The children's hospital'

An area of the playroom is set up with various items of hospital equipment, such as syringes without needles, bandages and dressings, stethoscopes, thermometers, tubing, teaspoons, masks, hats, aprons, gowns, pillows, blankets. The children are then invited to dress up and play at 'hospitals' together. The therapist may or may not be given a 'play' role by the children, but the therapist can sensitively encourage the children to share the experience of their own medical investigative or treatment procedure with each other. Thus the therapist may use the example of two children in the group playing at giving an injection to centre the attention of the group on this activity. The therapist will then encourage the group to describe their experiences and share the feelings aroused by such procedures. Clearly it is important to ensure that the play activity engaged in remains safe while retaining an entertaining and therapeutic quality.

CONCLUSIONS

1. By recreating hospital situations and experiences the children are given the opportunity to attempt to master the anxieties inherent in such situations.
2. By sharing the hospital procedures within a group the children are able to communicate their feelings and anxieties and with help from the therapist to seek mutual reassurance and support.
3. Painful and invasive procedures can be explored in the group in a way that reduces the trauma and anxiety of the actual experience. This can be followed up by the expectation of the child involved that he will receive accolade from his peer group after the event as well as further opportunity to talk to the group about his experience.

CHRONIC DISABILITY

We are referring here to conditions such as cystic fibrosis, renal problems and diabetes amongst others which, because the illness consists of remissions and relapses, sometimes necessitates hospital admission for treatment not only of the primary system affected but of other systems in the body which may be affected. Chronic physical illness is debilitating in every way. There may be physical restrictions to be observed, dietary instructions to be followed and medication to be taken. All of these serve as constant reminders to the child of the physical illness from which he suffers, and the extent to which he is able to adjust to this, and to accept and accommodate the condition yet learn to live and grow with it, will depend on the help that he receives from his family, friends, teachers and perhaps most importantly from the medical and nursing staff that he has contact with.

Frequent and repeated hospitalisation for these children can become obstacles to their growth and development. Thus for the child, for instance, who realises that his dependency needs can only be met when he is ill or in hospital, there develops a liking for hospital and its routine that can only be regarded as unhealthy. Obviously when hospitalisation is indicated it must be readily available to the child although it may be useful then to shorten the hospital admission and to use the time available to help the family and the child to learn to cope with the illness in other ways. Hospitals, on the other hand, can represent failure to those children and their families who have learned to accept their illness and yet strive to grow up normally. Hospital admission can also be very traumatic for those children and their families who engage in a denial of the illness and for whom hospitalisation brings back the reality of the condition that they would prefer to feel does not exist. Thus on the one hand the dependent child with a chronic physical illness may be admitted to hospital, and then seems to actually enjoy the experience of being in hospital while on the other hand a child may be admitted who feels angry, disappointed and who feels a failure. Both these kinds of children and their families need help in the task of acknowledging the reality of the problem and in being able to deal with it appropriately. For the children involved opportunities are available during the hospital stay to engage in group work to look at all of these issues in a helpful and monitoring way.

Making Masks

The children are asked to sit together in a circle. Each child is given three pieces of thin card large enough to cover their face. It is explained to the children that in the time allowed they are to make three masks, each one to represent the following:

1. How you feel in hospital.
2. How you feel at home.
3. How you feel at school.

It may be necessary to ask the children for some ideas to help them get started. For example, perhaps the mask may look angry, because he is in hospital, or sad because he is in hospital, etc. Allow a good range of art materials to allow self expression to develop.

When the masks are completed each child places one of their masks over their face and verbally expresses the meaning behind each of their masks. It may be useful to have a set phrase for each mask to encourage verbalisation:

At school I feel . . .
At home I feel . . .
At hospital I feel . . .

Following this exercise, a discussion takes place in which the participants are encouraged to elaborate on their own statements, as well as comment on each others' remarks and so to broaden the topic to feelings and coping mechanisms that each of the children may have developed with their own chronic disability.

CONCLUSIONS

1 By identifying specific feelings associated with hospital, with home and with school, feelings which may well be interchangeable, the child developed a measure of insight into the 'confusion' that may otherwise exist in which the prevailing emotion in all aspects of life is predominantly negative.
2 By sharing these feelings in a group, the children develop greater empathy for each other, feel less isolated in their own suffering and can identify with a group to whom they can hopefully turn for support.
3 In repeated exercises with variations on the same theme, an opportunity is presented for the child to express feelings of resentment, loss, guilt and frustration with comments from the group that can be supportive or comforting but overall constructive, in helping a peer come to terms with their particular disability.

ADDITIONAL EXERCISE

A further activity which will encourage children to externalise their feelings about life in hospital is by portraying their dreams or nightmares.

Dreams/nightmares

A suitable small group of children are brought together. The therapist explains to the children that during the night we often dream sometimes the dreams are nice and at other times they are frightening. This is particularly so when we are away from home. Each child is then given art materials to express a particular dream. At the end of the art period the dreams are shared with each other. If a child insists that he/she never dreams allow him/her to paint a picture 'a pretend dream'. The information in this picture will reflect the child's feelings and may be quite revealing.

HOSPITALS CAN BE QUITE NICE PLACES REALLY 79

CONCLUSIONS

1 Specific dreams/nightmares may reflect an unconscious working through of the child's fears and anxieties about hospitalisation, separation, or the trauma of the medical and surgical procedures involved.
2 By sharing these feelings a sense of relief is obtained, an element of reality is introduced to counter the fantasies and a generally supportive atmosphere is created for the child within the peer group and with the staff.

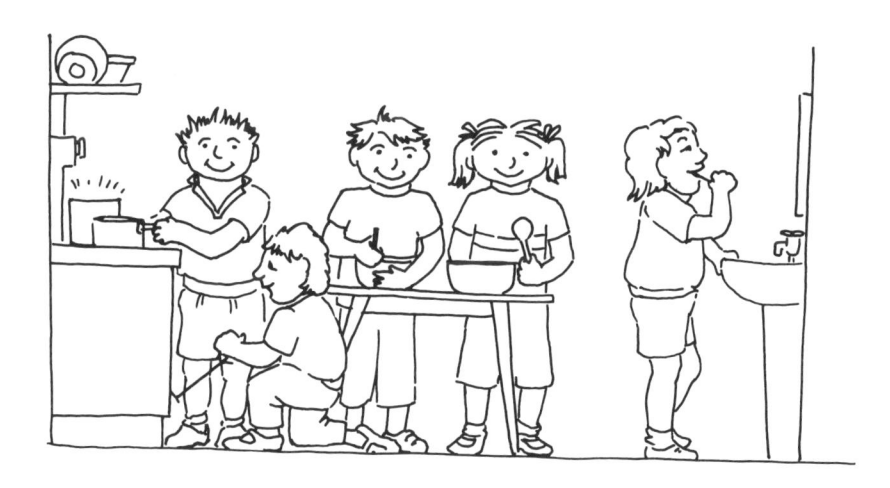

8 Coping with handicap

Handicap is a relative phenomenon in that the degree of handicap is determined by its deviation from the norm. The norm itself may be social or cultural, physical or mental, developmental or, for that matter, be any other parameter by which comparisons of people can be made. For the purpose of this chapter, we shall be looking at the concept of physical handicap and including in that category all those conditions in which the physical disability is present in a child of average intelligence or, at most, where a diagnosis of mild mental handicap is made. The reasons for establishing this requirement has to do with the authors' views on the feasibility of group work with children who have sufficient cognitive ability to make the group experience useful. Reference can be made to other chapters in this book, namely on 'physical awareness', 'social awareness' and 'the child in hospital', where issues arising in different kinds of handicap have been discussed and group exercises have been suggested.

Assessment, diagnosis and treatment of physical handicap is a task requiring a multi-disciplinary approach in which professionals from various disciplines pool their findings to provide a statement of the needs of the child and his family and recommend how best these needs can be met. The place of group work in such a scheme can be seen in the first instance as providing a continuous assessment process in which the personal, social and emotional growth of the child can be monitored, as can the effects of other interventions, such as the use of physical-aids, etc. Another function of the group would be to help prevent the development of secondary psycho-social difficulties and, of course, where these difficulties are already present the group experience may be useful in helping the child in their resolution.

Psychological Aspects of Physical Handicap

In talking about physical handicap, reference is being made to a wide variety of conditions as diverse as major motor disorder, such as cerebral palsy, to perceptual difficulties, such as poor hearing or vision, to chronic disability from, for example, cystic fibrosis or renal problems, to the minor albeit distressing problems, such as facial blemishes. Reference is also made to the manner in which these disabilities have come about, the significance of the way in which this has happened, and the age at which the disability makes itself known. Thus, there may be varying degrees of significance in the congenital or acquired conditions, or those resulting from trauma, as well as the ages at which these conditions become manifest.

In discussing the psychological aspects of physical handicap, it is important to know the interactive nature of the problem in terms of the relationship between physical handicap and psychological problems. Clearly not all physically handicapped children have psychological problems simply because they happen to be physically handicapped, just as, for example, many physically normal children may be maladjusted. It does appear to be the case though, that the stress of coping with the physical disability can predispose the development of psychological problems so that the physically handicapped children may well be at greater risk of having psychological problems. Again there may well be difficulties that exist independent of the disability itself such as, for example, family problems that become camouflaged by complaints about the physical handicap. The point being made here is that physical handicap becomes a ready target for displacement of other difficulties within the family as if it was not enough of a burden to carry in itself.

The physically handicapped child may live in a family in which sentiments are expressed that the child is keenly aware of. Parents have to come to terms with the loss of not having produced a perfect child; of having to cope with the problems of physically handicapped child in terms of the nurturing of that child that requires greater hard work without the same degree of satisfaction that one would expect from the normal child. Disappointment, resentment and frustration are experienced. Over-protection and over-indulgence may take place. Denial of the disability and to wish to view the child as normal may occur. Pushing the child to capitalise on existing potential, academic or otherwise, to compensate for the disability may also be a feature.

The attitude of the siblings is important in the extent to which they are accommodating or rejecting of the physically handicapped child. They may resent the greater attention that the physically handicapped child receives. They may resent the stigma attached to having a physically handicapped brother or sister.

The feelings that the child himself experiences will determine part of the interaction. These feelings are broadly outlined below as those of trust or lack of it, feelings of guilt and low self-esteem for children with congenital handicap. Feelings of loss for children who through some misfortune have an acquired handicap. Clearly there will be features common to children with all kinds of handicap and it must therefore be read in that context.

Before going to look at these feelings that the child experiences, a brief word about the use of group work with such children. As mentioned earlier, the authors feel that it is important from the point of view of the child receiving the maximum benefit from group work, that he should be of average intelligence or of a sufficient developmental level to be able to symbolise and think operationally. This is because concepts that we would hope to consider would require such a phase of development. Secondly, because physical handicap, again as mentioned earlier, requires an inter-disciplinary approach, it would be useful to involve other members of the team in group work and to report back to the team as a whole on the progress of a child in the group so that targets can be co-ordinated in the long term plans for care of the child. Finally, it is taken for granted that the physically handicapped child on his own may be helped in a group but it is important, where applicable, for parents as well to receive advice, help and support in the task of coming to terms with their own problems and in their task of looking after their child.

TRUST

For most physically handicapped children the process of assessment, diagnosis and treatment starts early in life. This usually implies investigative procedures in the context of hospitalisation during which time the children meet several adults who each seem to have an interest in one particular aspect of the child's development. Procedures may be painful and make the experience of separation while in hospital even more acute. The child has difficulty in making or sustaining relationships and may be confused by a wide variety of adults who, while caring and concerned, sometimes have to do painful and nasty things to the child. Trust becomes a key issue as the child grows older in his relationship with those around him. In the group situation the child may have difficulty in being able to trust other group members, or the group therapist enough to talk about unresolved feelings and fantasies. As such, unless this area is tackled first, the child may not be able to benefit from ongoing work in the group.

The following group experience is designed to enable group members to talk about and in some way enact their experiences of being able or not able to trust people close to them.

Concentric Circles

Each child is seated in a circle and is supplied with a piece of drawing paper and a pencil. In the middle of the paper the child places a dot to represent his or herself. The children are then asked to place concentric circles around the dot concerning the people they trust most and move outward to people they least trust. These people should include the family, people at the school or institution and other group members.

The drawings are then laid out on the floor for others to view. Questions should be encouraged but the therapist may need to help out important points and make similarities between trust issues.

CONCLUSIONS

1   This exercise will help the child identify in his own mind the people who are important and to the opposite extreme of trusting no one.
2   It will encourage the group to see that they may share similar feelings related to trust and this may lead to a starting point of building up trust within the group. This will then be helpful to further beneficial group sessions.

The next exercise based on trust is not necessarily to bring trust issues to the fore but more to help the group establish trust.

Blind Leading

It will depend on the disability of the individual as to how this exercise is carried out. If the children are ambient the exercise will include moving around the room, otherwise it can be carried out whilst seated. One child pairs up with another child and they agree amongst themselves who is going to shut their eyes and pretend they are blind. The other child is then responsible for leading the 'blind' child around and introducing him to different textures, different temperatures, different shapes, etc. If this exercise needs to be stationary then the 'sighted' child brings objects to the 'blind' child. After an agreed length of time the two children working together swop roles.

When the exercise is exhausted everyone sits together in a circle to discuss topics such as, how did you feel during the exercise?, what was it like to feel responsible for someone, did you feel safe being moved around blind, what senses did you use? etc.

CONCLUSIONS

1. This exercise encourages personal interaction through the sense of touch.
2. It encourages feedback regarding perception.
3. It allows trust to develop by having to assume responsibility for a person.
4. It allows the opportunity of discussing trust without directly focusing on the subject and therefore reducing defence barriers.

GUILT

The physically handicapped child becomes aware quite early in life of the extra attention that is required of those around him to meet his needs. Thus he is fussed over more so than his siblings and things are made 'easier' for him. Along with this awareness, a second sense develops of a certain despair or frustration in the family that vaguely relates to his own helplessness. This feeling becomes more acute as time goes by and may, in fact, be spelt out in no uncertain terms by sibs or parents. The family lifestyle becomes restricted on the child's account and the child feels and is sometimes made to feel responsible for this state of affairs. Feelings of guilt emerge for causing problems to others. Questions begin to come as to why the child is suffering in this way. In a world where introspection can be only too readily resorted to, the child may by now be blaming himself for the condition that he finds himself in. Fantasies may occur in terms of this being some kind of retribution for major sins committed in the past. The child may not feel free, with feelings of guilt, to achieve, progress, or in any way allow himself a chance to develop opportuniies to the full.

COPING WITH HANDICAP 85

EXERCISE 1

This exercise is designed to help relieve the child of some of the fantasies of guilt that he may carry around with him and which makes life more difficult than it need be.

The group leader presents the group with a large sheet of paper on which is drawn a large pair of scales. One side of the scales is marked positive. The sheet of paper is affixed to the wall or notice-board. The children are then given three small slips of paper on which they are asked to write down good things about themselves in relation to family life. Examples can be given, such as 'I am helpful around the house', 'I am generally cheerful', etc. When each child has completed the task, they place the slips of paper into a cardboard box. The children are then invited to pick out slips of paper from the box and to stick or pin them on the side of the scales marked positive. It soon becomes clear that there is an imbalance with a lot of positive suggestions and nothing on the other. The child may comment on this and the group leader invites the children to write down on one slip of paper something about themselves that they do not find particularly helpful. An example may be provided, 'I am often sulky'. The procedure is repeated as for the positive suggestions, and the new slips of paper are pinned onto the other side of the scales. A discussion is encouraged to allow the children to comment on the statements that have been made.

CONCLUSIONS

1 A sense of proportion is created in terms of the positive and not so positive contributions that each child makes to family life.
2 An idea conveyed that it is acceptable to have 'good' and 'bad' bits in everyone.
3 The reality of the weighing up process challenges some of the fantasies that the child may hold about his role in contributing to problems of family life.
4 Group discussions allow the children to share their fears and anxieties, to have these commented upon by peers, and this creates a sense of togetherness.
5 A deliberate attempt is made to engender more positive than negative suggestions, both to reflect the truth of the situation as well as to leave the group feeling better about themselves.

LOW SELF-ESTEEM

In a world where 'body worship' sometimes assumes cult proportions, it is not surprising that the physically handicapped child feels inferior, ashamed, envious or self-pitying from having a poor body image. In many instances, these feelings have been reinforced by throwaway remarks or comments borne of frustration and disappointment from those who look after the physically disabled child. In other cases the child may have experienced excessive over-protection and indulgence to the point where the child is ill-equipped to relate to his peers on an equal and sharing basis, and consequently suffers. Inadequate models for imitation and identification further inhibit the child from testing out his own capabilities and he may well be left with a feeling that he is unable to achieve what he would like.

The following group exercise looks at the possibility of using peer group approval to make the child view himself more constructively and hence more positively.

Encounter

Initially the children sit round in a circle. They are given a piece of paper and pen to write down what they feel are their good characteristics and what they feel are their bad characteristics.

The papers are then folded and left to one side. The next stage is for the group leader to pin a piece of paper to each person's back and on this each participant must write a short description of the person whose back they are writing on.

The last stage is to come back together and for the children to have retrieved and to read out aloud the positive descriptions others have made of them and encourage them to share their own initial private writings.

CONCLUSIONS

1   Initially the children are made to think about themselves which will help to increase their own self awareness.
2   The information they receive from each other will help to increase their self-esteem by the nature of such positive feedback.
3   The children will have to interact with each other and therefore encourage recognition, co-operation and awareness of others.
4   As the children share information they will begin to gain more trust.

COPING WITH HANDICAP

The next exercise again is useful to help the child think constructively about himself.

Coat of Arms

Seated in a circle each group member is asked to copy the shield as drawn below. The individual is then asked to fill in each space as appropriate, using pictures, symbols and words. At the end each person talks about their shield and explains what they have drawn.

MOTTO	
A HAPPY MEMORY	A SAD MEMORY
A WISH FOR ONE YEAR	WHAT WILL YOU BE DOING IN FIVE YEARS TIME

This activity can be done on an individual basis or as a group activity where the shield is done by the group members working together to produce an end product upon which they agree.

CONCLUSIONS

1 It is a good way of establishing a rapport and getting to know the children's feelings.

2 The child has to commit his feeling on paper, thinking not only of now but looking ahead to the future.
3 If done as a group task the children must interact, developing social awareness and group cohesiveness.
4 If done on an individual basis the group later enters into a discussion about each other's motto, therefore creating awareness of others.

LOSS

The previously healthy child at school who loses a limb, or an eye, or some function of the body, goes through a period of mourning for the lost part. Adjustments are made to the new circumstances and abilities. The period of grief gives way to feelings of acceptance and then to constructive appraisal of the future. In many instances this process becomes obstructed at various points of the grief process. Thus the disability may be denied, blame may be attributed, the child may blame himself, the child may become depressed. Disinterest may follow despite the efforts of the professionals to help him. In all of these obstacles to resolution of the grief, the child may be unknowingly encouraged by his near and dear ones who may find it hard to accept the loss themselves, may deny that it has occurred and may adopt a litigious stance against the perpetrators of the event or against hospital staff for not doing more for the child.

The following group exercise may be useful in helping children who have suffered a grievous loss come to terms with their disability.

The Secret Box

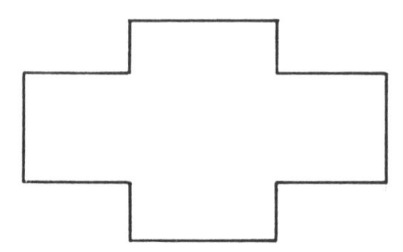

The children are seated around in a circle and are supplied with paper, pencils and scissors. The children are asked to cut out the following shape, which can be folded into a box. For the younger and less dextrous child, a previously made template could be used to draw around. Before assembling the box, on the inside they write their feelings which they hide from others, and on the outside of the box they write how they think other people see them. When the box is assembled the children come together and show their boxes. The group must make a decision if their hidden feelings are shared, but the group is allowed to comment on how other children think they are perceived.

CONCLUSIONS

1. The box will capture the child's imagination and be a useful way to help them express their feelings on their disabilities.
2. The sharing of feelings will increase their own self awareness and that of others.
3. The children will gain some strength from each other, because each child will have suffered some loss due to their disability.
4. The group leader will be made more aware of the child's perception of his/her disability and can use this information in a positive way.

9 Groups on the school timetable

It perhaps goes without saying that teachers go in for teaching because they are interested in children. This interest extends beyond mere pursuit of the curriculum to include an active interest in the child's welfare, his development and his well-being. The teacher/child relationship is often a precious entity and one which fosters trust and confidence so that it is not uncommon to hear of children who have confided private and important information to their teachers in the first instance rather than to anybody else. The school system itself is geared to providing for the child's overall needs to include his educational, social and emotional needs. The upshot of this is that for the majority of children, who on average spend some fifteen thousand hours at school, the experience of school life is often remembered as a happy and fulfilling time. There are, however, a minority of children for whom this is not the case and it is to the needs of these children that this chapter attempts to address itself.

We are talking here about the disruptive child, the withdrawn child, the truant, the school refuser, the child with specific learning difficulties, the under-achieving child, and the child who is unable to form satisfactory relationships within the peer group. Who looks after the needs of these children? Are there identified resources outside of school which can be called upon to help the children with these difficulties? The practice varies enormously between schools and this is determined, not least, by the prevailing ethos and atmosphere within the school. Thus, marked differences can be observed between schools in close geographical proximity, and taking pupils from similar catchment populations, in terms of the rate and type of difficulties that children present with. Of the problems that do arise, some schools may, in their wish to be self-sufficient, offer a variety of programmes to help their children in difficulty. Others may prefer to use the referral process to child guidance clinics and hospital departments of child psychiatry. Other factors, such as availability of expertise of psychiatrists, psychologists (educational and clinical), social workers and others, and the willingness of these people to work 'on site' (in school), or their preference only to do so at their respective bases, will determine the nature and type of help that the school and the child receives.

Of the options available, the most appropriate choice in the event of the school requiring outside help is for the professions concerned to work on site, namely in school itself, and in active liaison with the staff in helping and advising on children in difficulties. Of the treatment options available, the first choice would be for the use of group work in tackling the problems described. The rationale for the choices made is based, firstly, on the idea that children would best be helped in their own environment and, secondly, that many of the problems that arise are a direct reflection of difficulties in group relationships. Clearly there will be cases that do require referral to outside agencies in order to provide other kinds of therapies that may be indicated.

As far as group work in schools is concerned, it is important that the practicalities are examined if the idea is to materialise. Many factors, including staffing levels and time-tabling, militate against the idea. But again it is possible, as some schools who do practise in this way will maintain, that with a little ingenuity and a lot of motivation the problem is surmountable. Obviously, this is easier said than done and a project such as this will require considerable discussion, as well as goodwill on the part of those concerned. Again, practice will vary in terms of the type of group offered, numbers of children per group, etc. As a general guideline, we would suggest mixed groups, that is children presenting with different types of problems, both sexes or single-sexed, six to eight per group, and running for five to ten hourly sessions held on a weekly basis.

For purposes of clarification, we are talking here of the needs of primary school children, although it is hoped that some of the ideas developed would apply equally to secondary schools, with certain obvious exceptions relating to issues emerging in early or middle adolescence.

We shall now look at problems relating to the school refusing child, and the child who poses a 'problem' in the classroom and the playground. Of the latter, there are two categories, the first being the child who is socially isolated from his peers, and the second being the child who is socially integrated with a sub-group of children who pose similar problems.

THE SCHOOL REFUSER

The term 'school refuser' is perhaps a misnomer in that school refusal in the primary school child does not equate with the clinical picture that is sometimes seen in the middle adolescent period. The commonest problem occurring in primary school applies to children in first year. It is common enough for children going to school for the first time to be apprehensive about the new and strange environment. Many schools have taken this into account and allow a parent to accompany the child into the classroom and, in some instances, allow the parent to stay with the child, if necessary, for the duration of the school time for up to a week or more. Most will have acclimatised by this time, although some children continue to have difficulties in separating from the parent (and vice versa) and this can be a stressful experience for both child and adult. The second type of situation in which there is a reluctance to attend school can arise from a variety of precipitating factors. Thus, the child who has been absent through illness, brief or prolonged, may become anxious about attending school for fear of having fallen behind in work or having lost his place in the ever changing group dynamic. The same would apply to the child who is experiencing difficulties in the peer group, or with the teachers, or to the child who has learning difficulties or even to the bright and over-competitive child who is obsessively concerned with perfection. The third type of refusal relates to problems in the home and ranges from the child being kept home to the child insisting on staying at home to ensure that his fears about parental break up do not materialise, or to ensure that his fantasies of returning to an empty home, where there has been parental strife, should not be realised.

For all these children, the school becomes a threatening environment from which they prefer to stay away. It is important, therefore, to understand for each child the problems that have caused them to be anxious and in addition to be reassuring, encouraging and supportive, as well as to seek expert help where necessary.

The following exercise will use available materials (plasticine and play-doh) to explore feelings about the transition from home to school.

'Modelling the Environment'

The children (preferably in a small group) are asked to use the plasticine/play-doh to make models of their homes. When the children have completed this step, the houses are placed together on a large sheet of paper. Once the houses are set out, roads, streets, perhaps school, parks, etc, can be drawn onto the sheet. When the task is completed, the children should be encouraged to sit around in a group and talk freely about home life and how it is different or similar to school life. To encourage discussion, the teacher may ask the children things such as how long does it take to reach school; what time does everyone get up to get ready for school; who travels on the bus or in a car; who takes

GROUPS ON THE SCHOOL TIMETABLE 93

the child to school; questions which will help the child to become aware of their feelings about having to leave home and come to school.

CONCLUSIONS

1 By taking the theme 'home', the teacher is helping the children to realise that home is important and will still be there after school.
2 Each child models their own house and, therefore, is saying to the other children that we are 'all in the same boat'. Hence the children are gaining peer awareness and group identity.
3 The children are encouraged to become aware of their feelings about separating from parents.
4 By becoming involved in their task the children are starting to settle, be involved, interact with their peers, and accept the adult.
5 The use of plasticine/play-doh is a familiar material which reduces feelings of anxiety or threat.

This exercise can be used in the same way as 'Modelling the Environment'.

'Home Collage'

The leader prepare sheets of paper with a basic drawing of a house showing internal rooms.

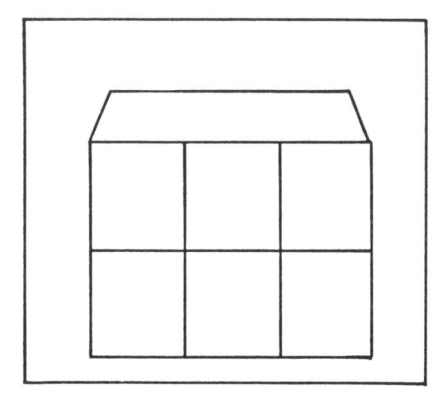

The children are seated together as a group and given a sheet of prepared paper. A wide range of materials should be available such as paints, felt-tip pens and collage materials. The leader explains that each child fills in the home diagram relating it to their own home. People may be added as well as material objects.

The picture, when completed, should be shared with the group and a group discussion, as in the previous exercise, should be encouraged.

THE 'PROBLEM' CHILD IN THE CLASSROOM AND IN THE PLAYGROUND

The commonest cause for referral of a child by the school to outside agencies is misbehaviour within the school premises. The problem can arise in the classroom where a child or group of children may distract other pupils or challenge the authority of the teacher. Problems can occur in the school playground where there may be fighting, bullying or scapegoating. In addition to this, there may be isolated incidents of stealing or destructive behaviour resulting in damage to school property.

Why does this occur, who are the children responsible, and what can be done to help the situation? It is generally agreed that schools maintain, necessarily so, a regimented environment. Infringement of the rules is not easily tolerated, at least not when it becomes repetitive. Teachers come to represent adult authority figures on a par with a substitute parental status. This is a given authority that accompanies the teaching role. There is also the personal authority of the teacher as an individual and the picture is completed with the teacher bringing to his work his own personality, likes and dislikes.

The child who misbehaves consistently, violates the code of the system and that of its operators. There are several ways in which the system itself may generate or contribute to this state of affairs, but we are concerned here with the child and his motives for interacting with the school in this inappropriate way.

We shall now go on to look at the two categories of children mentioned earlier who may give cause for concern.

THE SOCIALLY ISOLATED CHILD

This child draws attention to himself in the classroom by clowning or by acts of bravado in challenging the authority of the teacher. In the playground he can be interfering, invite bullying and scapegoating, steal apparently unnecessarily or engage in destructive behaviour. The premise for all of this is simply that some kind of attention is better than none even if this attention is negative and punitive from his peers and teachers. This child suffers from chronically poor self-esteem for reasons that range from low achievement to social ineptitude. He may have some physical deformity that sets him apart, or specific learning difficulties that keep him from doing as well as he might. More usually he may come from a family with intense rivalry in the sibship where negative behaviour becomes reinforced in its elicting negative attention. The child may come from a family where he does not feel good enough. The teacher may come to represent a depriving, uncaring and hostile figure.

The problem with all such children is that the undesired behaviour has multiple causation. An instinctive response may be to refer the child for 'expert' help. This in the knowledge that the same child poses no problems at all and, in fact, flourishes when attended on a one-to-one basis. But then the argument goes that if the child has a difficulty in sharing, should he not learn or be taught that this is an essential part of life experience or, for that matter, that schools and teachers cannot afford the luxury of providing such children with the individual input they may need.

The following exercise is aimed at exploring the underlying reasons for the child's unacceptable behaviour.

'I Would Like to Be . . .'

The teacher sets out a variety of items which are available in the classroom, e.g. chalk, blocks, shapes, cars, people, model animals, board dusters, elastic band and paper clip. There should be more items than children. The children are then asked to choose an item and with pen and paper write about themselves as the item. The opening line would read, 'I would like to be . . .'

For example, on one occasion, when this exercise was used with a group of children, a nine-year-old girl who was said to be disruptive in class chose a red piece of fur fabric. Her story began, I would like to be a piece of red fur fabric, because red is a very bright colour. I wish I was bright. I would like to be made of fur. Everyone strokes fur. This girl's problems had started since the arrival of a baby brother. The exercise demonstrated that she needed to re-establish her position in the family and gain some positive attention.

When all the children have finished writing they should be encouraged to share their ideas with each other. The teacher could do the exercise alongside the children and when it comes to discussion time the teacher could share his ideas first as a model for the children. The involvement of the teacher on this level helps the children feel more relaxed about releasing and sharing feelings.

CONCLUSIONS

1. The material for the exercise is available in the classroom so that the exercise is easily organised.
2. The exercise is like a classroom activitiy
3. The children can indulge in creative expression through the projection of themselves into an object. This will help the teacher gain understanding of the child and help the child gain insight of himself, allowing an opportunity for change.
4. If the teacher joins in the activity the children may feel less anxious about discussing things on a more personal level.
5. By being projective the activity camouflages the fact that it explores personal feelings, allowing the children to be open and direct.
6. Children sharing the activity may be able to gain some understanding of how each other feels.

NB: If this activity is used for the younger children who have not yet mastered writing, it can be turned into a verbal exercise. It would be better to use it in small groups. This will allow time to focus on each child.

The next exercise explores more of the child's own self-image.

'Things I Do'

The group sits in a circle. The leader explains that they are all going to take turns to complete sentences. The first sentence is something which they do badly—'I am very bad at doing . . .'

The leader should start the round to set an example and will consequently start the next two. The second sentence is something people tell them off about—'I am told off for . . .' The third sentence is something which they do well—'I am very good at . . .' The fourth sentence is something people tell them they do well—'I am praised for . . .'

Each round can lead into a discussion or the discussion could be saved until the end. However, the discussion is important to seize and check out statements which have been made.

CONCLUSIONS

1. Each person is allowed to say what they feel without comment.
2. Everyone is given an equal chance of saying what they feel and, therefore, there is no hierarchy.

3   The leader will be able to use the information sensitively to help a child gain further insight either about himself or others.
4   Sharing of information creates a feeling of togetherness and identity.

THE SOCIALLY INTEGRATED CHILD

This child identifies with a sub-group of children who are part of a sub-culture of society that has its own value systems. Some would describe this child as being vulnerable to or, in fact, pre-delinquent. This is too much of a generalisation and perhaps what is really meant here is that there must be something wrong with the child and his family if between them they do not place the same emphasis on education and the educational system as the more academically aspiring of their peers and teachers. Other arguments prevail that have perhaps a greater validity and to which there are political, economic and social overtones. In practice this child is disruptive in the classroom at the behest of and along with two or three other like-minded children. Again, as with the socially isolated child, the reasons for this behaviour are various but more likely to be social than emotional. The child may come from a family with poor modelling, inconsistent discipline, disregard for authority and a devaluing of educational aspirations. In short, the child is poorly socialised in a conventional sense, and the fear is that this may also manifest in areas outwith the school.

The problem is that it is only too easy to be dismissive of the child and his family given the arguments above. It may be felt that, short of major educational and curriculum overhaul and sweeping social change, little can be achieved. Again this is the sort of generalisation that is untrue. If anything, there are always indicators from the child and his family that they would wish to be helpful if help was forthcoming. After all, the school is a powerful system and failure to conform with the system brings its own stress that the child and family would wish to avoid rather than invite.

There are many exercises which develop social skills. We have chosen the following exercise which will help to build up self-esteem and confidence with the peer group.

'Gifts'

Divide the class into small groups of children. The disruptive sub-group should be split among different groups. Hand out sheets of paper to each group and ask each individual to take a sheet and tear the piece into the same number of pieces as there are children in the group. On each slip the child should write the name of another child in the group and a gift he would like to give to that child so that all the members of the group have a gift. Stress that it is important to think about the person the gift is for, and that these gifts should be appropriate, personal and different for each of the children. When everyone in the group is finished, everyone passes their slips of paper to the appropriate children. Each child will end up with a number of gifts. One by one the children read out the gifts and try to identify the giver. Depending on the cohesiveness of the group, it would be useful to discover why certain gifts have been chosen.

CONCLUSIONS

1 A child whose behaviour is anti-social joins in with children who are more socially aware, thus allowing them a new experience.
2 By interacting with a small group, confidence will be built up.
3 Receiving gifts promotes a positive feeling and helps to boost self-esteem.
4 The gifts are a measure of the impression each child makes on each other. Therefore, some insight can be gained from the choice of gift.
5 Sharing verbal information will add clarity to the reasons behind giving a particular gift.

Describe a Diagram

Prepare some cards with simple diagrams on them, for example:

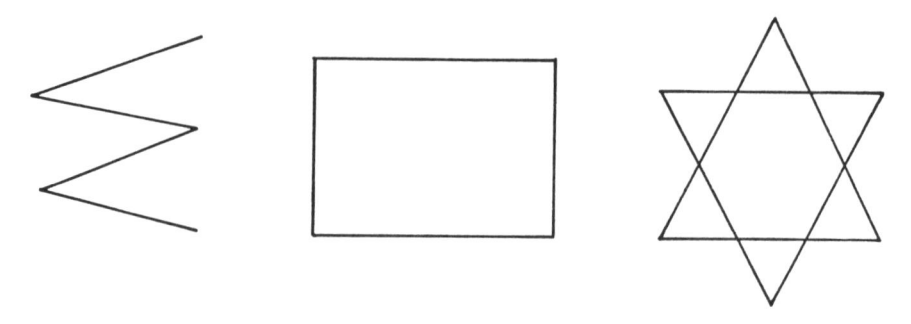

Explain that a volunteer is required to describe a diagram to the other children following one of the cards. From the description the other children draw what they hear, until the description is complete. The describer must not say anything as obvious such as draw a square. Each line must be treated separately. When the description and drawings are complete, they are all placed on the floor to view. Some results can be quite amazing.

CONCLUSIONS

1. Each child is given the opportunity to lead the group in a positive, therapeutic way. The response from the others will help to increase self-esteem.
2. Everyone plays a part and even the more difficult child is seen to interact, and therefore become more acceptable within the peer group.
3. The activity usually receives an amazing end, therefore helping the children to relax and enjoy the situation.

10 We live in groups—*residential schools*

The residential school placement is one of a set of positive therapeutic options available for the child who is unable to cope with the system or for the system that is unable to cope with the child. The system in this context is represented by the child's family, his school and the community in which he lives. Inability to cope with the system refers to difficulties in relationships between the child, his family and society. The residential school placement is referred to as a positive therapeutic option because it offers the opportunity of repairing some of these relationships by providing an alternative living system within which the child can be helped to become better equipped socially and emotionally to cope with the demands of the outside world.

The residential school is staffed by parent figures, viz. the teachers and the residential social workers. These people, along with the domestic, catering and maintenance staff, also represent the adults in society that the child has come across in the past and will meet in the future. The other occupants of the school, the children, represent both the peer group as well as, and perhaps more importantly, the sibling group. The school itself becomes for the child a little world with its own ethos and value system. Although contact with the child's family is maintained through weekends and holidays spent at home, the school remains the place where the child has a major social and emotional investment.

The process of arriving at a residential school placement is long and complicated. It involves assessment and treatment of the child and family, case conferences and inter-agency negotiations, placement discussions and placement finding battles. It is a process that if often fraught and marked with uncertainty. For both the child and his family as well as for the helping agencies involved, the final reality of the residential school placement comes as a relief albeit tinged with sadness in the knowledge that the child is to be separated from his family, and guilt in the feeling that the child has somehow been failed by its helpers. It is time now for the 'alternative system' to take over the care of the child while retaining links and activity liaising with the referring agencies for the duration of the child's stay in the school and until his eventual return home.

In the following paragraphs we shall be looking at some of the difficulties that the child will encounter during his stay at residential school. Group exercises are suggested that will go some way towards helping the child cope with these difficulties. Five areas will be looked at, i.e. the settling in phase, coping with feelings of rejection, getting on with the peer group, relating to staff, and the return to the family.

THE SETTLING IN PHASE

From the point that the child first steps into the residential school he will be entering a new 'mini society' and like all new experiences this can be a strange and wonderful or strange and terrifying. It is likely in fact to be a mixture of both. Many of these children have experienced a near total breakdown of relationships with their families and will be looking forward to starting afresh with a new set of adults, a new set of peers and a new 'home' to live in. At the same time there will be a strong feeling of loss and being 'lost' in this new environment with its rules, its regulations and its expectations. The child 'knows' nobody. With help he will learn to find his way around the building and its grounds, and to learn the timetable. These are the least of his problems. First impressions are often lasting and the child will be seeking to make the acceptable impression. He will place himself on the lowest rung of the pecking order in the peer group and wait to be invited to climb the social ladder. With the adults he will be cagey, to say the least! Trust is the sort of luxury he cannot, for the moment, afford. He will be gauging responses to his overtures and will react accordingly. It is altogether a difficult and trying time for the child and is marked by conflicting emotions of sadness and anger at his loss, of anxiety and apprenshion about the present and the future but also, and quite importantly so, of an eagerness and a need to succeed in his new setting. Clearly it is essential to capitalise on this latter urge while acknowledging and working with all the other feelings that the child is experiencing.

The following exercise allows the child an opportunity to get to know his peer group better. It would be used at the beginning of the group and thereby act as a 'warm up' exercise.

'Name find'

Each group member is given a pen and piece of paper on which to write their own name or if they prefer their nickname and another piece of paper for collecting names. Their name is pinned to their sleeve. The children are then expected to mill around rapidly rather than slowly. The object of the exercise is to make a list of everyone's name. When a number of lists are completed the group sits down together and each member tells everyone their name. By the end of the exercise even the ones who did not complete their list will have been made familiar with the group.

CONCLUSIONS

1. The exercise encourages physical activity and will therefore help to reduce tension and anxiety.
2. There is the opportunity to break down 'icy' social barriers within the peer group, by focusing on a task.
3. Each group member is given the same task, therefore everyone is treated as equal.
4. At the end of the exercise everyone will have met and some names will be remembered.

'Family Names'

Pieces of paper are prepared with family names (one family member per slip of paper), Mother Buttan, Father Buttan, Sister Buttan, Baby Buttan. Each person receives a name and then moves around the room swopping their names, with anyone they meet. When the leader shouts 'STOP' everyone yells out their family name and try to link up with their family. The family group must sit on top of each other in the following order—Father, Mother, Sister and Baby. The aim is to try to be seated as a family first. Swop family papers and start again.

CONCLUSIONS

As for 'Name find' but there is no focus on learing each others names, but the nature of the exercise will allow the children to get to know each other better.

FEELING REJECTED

Long before the child has been 'officially' told of the decision to be placed at a residential school, he will have picked up the idea that such a move was on the cards. He will have been at the centre of numerous family rows and arguments concerning his behaviour at home or at school. He will blame himself for causing the family concern. He may begin to entertain the idea idea that the family will be better off if he were 'put away'. This would be reinforced by hints and open threats from the parents that they would wish him out of the home. The child is confused in that try as he may, the problems continue and he can only conclude that he is bad and therefore deserves what is coming to him. The family, unable to see the wood for the trees, collude with this image that the child has of himself. Helping agencies endeavour, with or without success, to clarify the family dynamics and to bring a sense of reality to the actual causes of problems in the family. In the event of failure the point arrives where threat becomes fact because it is clear that both child and family are locked in stalemate and that alternative solutions are called for. This rationality is perhaps understood and accepted by the parents but really means very little to the child. The reality for the child is that he is bad enough to have to leave the home. The other reality is that, much as he might have hoped that the family would continue to want him despite everything, the fact is that they do not. The shunned fantasy of rejection becomes reality.

The following exercise helps to explore the feelings behind rejection.

'Face collage'

With the group seated in a circle make a list with them of all the different emotions they can think of. Some children may have difficulty with the meaning of the word 'emotions' therefore ask someone in the group to explain its meaning.

The making of the list is to warm the child up for the second part of the exercise.

The second part consists of asking the children to work together and make a collage of faces cut out from magazines. The faces should represent all the emotions which have previously been suggested. The cut out faces are to be arranged and glued onto a large sheet of paper. It is important each member contributes some cut out faces.

When the collage is finished fix it onto the wall for all to see. The leader then takes the initiative to start finding out about the facial expressions promoting group discussion. The discussion can be steered towards more personal feelings particularly about rejection which is related to being at residential school.

CONCLUSIONS

1 The collage is a group product. This will help the individual within the group to feel safe, secure and with a place to belong.
2 Group co-operation and interaction is expected from the group. A feeling of group cohesion and sharing will build up.
3 The exercise encourages a release of a wide range of emotions.
4 It also encourages sharing of emotional feelings that are relevant to the child, and also awareness of how others are feeling.

EXERCISE I

'Opposite Emotions'

The group is divided into two groups. Each group sits in a line facing the other group. One group have to think of an emotion, e.g. anger, happiness, sadness, and mime this to the other group. The opposite group decide amongst themselves what the mime is and mime back the opposite emotion.

Once the two emotions have been recognised fully the group come together as a whole and discuss the feelings behind the emotions. Then the recipient groups starts an emotional mime.

CONCLUSIONS

1 Working in small groups will give some opportunity to get to know others in a less threatening way.
2 Again the focus of the activity is concerned with emotions and this gives the opportunity for discussion.
3 The ultimate aim of the group is to help the children express themselves particularly regarding feelings of rejection, therefore by sharing information group trust should develop.

GETTING ON IN THE PEER GROUP

The response of the peer group to the newcomer is always guarded and suspicious. This, after all, is a potential usurper, who has arrived to challenge the group for position and favour. He will also be demanding his share of time, affection and support from the staff. This in a situation where there are already too many mouths to feed and too little to feed them with. Let us assume that the newcomer is now an established member of the group. Does the scenario change? It does not. The jostling goes on for position and favour in the group and for position and favour with the staff. Within the peer group the interactions that take place are described in the Chapter on Social Awareness along with group exercises designed to help out some of the difficulties that arise. Within the context of the group—staff interaction and merely as an aside it is interesting to observe how the group behaviour, amiable or otherwise, tends to mirror the goings on within the staff group itself. For the main part, however, the staff contribution to group harmony is derived from the children's perceptions of staff fairness and justice in all circumstances and to all children. Where it is clear that all the children are held in equal regard and that attempts to win a special place by subterfuge is unnecessary. Many of these children will have come from families where the sibling rivalry stakes were high and they were the losers. These children will attempt to recoup their losses, starting on the premise that all adults like their parents, are unfair. It is important that the staff demonstrate otherwise and so prevent a repetition for the children of what occurred before. This will obviously require a knowledge of the child's individual and family history but then it is likely that there will be a common theme running through the history of most of the children in the school.

The following exercise will encourage the peer group to participate, interact together and have some fun.

'Polio'

One person in the group volunteers to be 'it'. The rest of the group work together. 'It' stands at one end of the room and the group stand at the other. The distance between the 'it' and the group should be a suitable distance to run. 'It' shouts out a theme such as foods, trees, cars, clothes to the others. They then huddle together to decide what item from the theme they will be. For example, if the theme is trees one group member may be an oak, another a beech, another a willow and so on. Someone in the group will shout out all the items to 'it'. 'It' replies by shouting out one of the group items. This immediately means action. If, for instance, oak was chosen, oak and 'it' must run and change place. Whoever is in place first will be the next 'it'. Although this exercise may sound complicated it is often known to children as a 'playground' game. The leader may decide to allow 'it' a limited number of goes to ensure everyone had a turn at 'it'.

CONCLUSIONS

1. Each group member takes a turn at 'it'. This is an opportunity to take a therapeutic leadership role.
2. The group have to work together, co-operating and making decisions.
3. The exercise allows positive group interaction.
4. They physical activity reduces any tension or anxiety which may be around.

EXERCIE 2

'Wave the Ocean'

Chairs are placed in a circle. When everyone is seated there should be two empty ones left over. Someone then volunteers to stand in the middle and issues one of the following commands: 'Wave to the left' and 'Wave to the right'. The whole group must move either to the left or the right in a sitting position. The person in the middle tries to sit on a chair and when he/she succeeds the person on his or her left takes the centre position, and the game continues.

CONCLUSIONS

1. The peer group are together and working as a whole. This should help them to feel more relaxed and at ease with their situation.
2. Although one person at a time is the focal point when the exercise is moving they should not feel self-conscious because the emphasis is on the physical activity. However, each individual is given the chance to be a leader.
3. The speed and concentration of the exercise will reduce anxiety and tension.

4   This is a good 'Warm Up' exercise to enable further positive group work to take place.

RELATING TO STAFF

The staff in residential schools work at different levels of responsibility and accountability in the school hierarchy. This can be quite confusing for the child who will have been introduced to the house parent, the senior house parent, the principal residential social worker and then to the teachers, the deputy and the headmaster. The one person that the child will relate most closely to, will be the key worker. This relationship will be, in the first instance, an immediate reflection of the child's relationship with his parents. The key worker is invariably in a close relationship with more than one child and the perennial issues of rivalry and jealousy are just some of the problems that have to be coped with. It is certainly helpful that the child comes into contact with several adults during the course of the day who will each be responsible for the same aspects of the child's welfare. This allows the child to make an emotional investment of varying degree and type in relationships with different members of staff. What does tend to happen at times though, is that the child can assume a position of power in being able to split or distort the perception of different staff members towards himself. Thus at case review for example, one often hears conflicting reports about the same child and it becomes important for the staff to understand how the child can and sometimes needs to, identify and relate to members of staff as good, bad or indifferent. Some of this may well be unconsciously allowed to happen by staff. More often than not, however, this kind of situation arises most frequently where there is inadequate staff communication or where there are problems in the school in the course of which staff differences reflect the parental differences and ways of handling that the child had already experienced in his home. For the purposes of this section it may be useful to focus on the problems arising from the child testing out the staff on the issue of caring, a subject that he has become intensely suspicious of.

The following exercise will encourage the child to look closely at his support system and the emotional investment linked to the system.

'Support systems'

Start with the group seated in a circle. Explain to them that they have to think about people (house parent, senior house parent, social worker, teachers, domestics, own peers) that are important to them within the residential school. The people may be valuable because they help with loneliness, sadness, confusion, anger, general conversation or entertainment. Magazines are then given out and each child is asked to cut out pictures that represent these people and a picture to represent him or herself. Likeness is not important. This picture representing the child is glued onto the centre of a sheet of paper. The rest of the people are place around 'self'. If someone is very close their picture will be near to 'self' if someone is not so close their picture will be placed at a distance from 'self'.

The exercise will finish with the sharing of pictures and explanations of who is who and what they represent.

CONCLUSIONS

1 The exercise is for each individual child to identify his support system within school.
2 It encourages awareness of other children's support systems and the importance of recognising other children's needs.
3 It raises the issue of how two or more children can satisfactorily 'shape' the attention of a particular member of staff and of how the group as a whole has to learn 'to make do' with the available staff resources.'

'Support Statements'

Ask each child to write down a statement about someone in the school who is supportive towards them. Then they must find a partner and together compromise their statements making one statement. Next they join another pair and do the same. This continues until the whole group are working together to produce one complete statement. When this is completed a general discussion should emerge as to what is behind the meaning of the statement and which people it is aimed at.

RETURN TO THE FAMILY

The child who has been given a 'leaving date' is held in high regard by his peers. He has made it. The child has that same eager but anxious anticipation that he experienced on first joining the school. There will also be the same sense of loss of peers and caring adults that he is leaving behind and it is important for the child to be able to acknowledge this.

Re-entering society as it were, is a difficult business and the child needs all the help he can get to achieve this successfully. In the first instance regular and frequent contact will have been maintained between the child and his family through weekends and holidays spent at home, from parents visiting the school and from school staff working with the family and child to try and resolve relationship difficulties. Next, there will be concrete arrangements made for future educational placement and for continuing professional social or psychological help where needed. At the same time there will be a recognition of the strong emotions surfacing within the child that are associated with leaving one 'family' and the uncertainty of entering another. The child's fear of alienation, of having lost his place in the family, of being unwelcome by his parents and siblings because he is a trouble-maker. All of these feelings will be reflected in the child's behaviour in the time that he has left in the school. This will range from sadness, to supposed indifference, to anger and protest at leaving, again, much in the same vein as occurred when he was leaving his family to come to residential school. The difference is, and it is a very important difference, that the child must be able to leave the school with the feeling of having a 'good' experience. This is often not something that is easily apparent in the child or readily expressed or for that matter even possible in the immediate turmoil of leaving. Nevertheless, with proper handling along the lines mentioned, it is possible for the child to be able to look back in the months and years ahead, at his time in residential school as having been a good and valuable experience.

The following exercise is one we often use when a child is leaving the group and moving back home. It always seems to provide a good leaving atmosphere. It needs to be the last exercise the group will do together.

'Positive suggestion'

The child who is leaving is the focus. The leader explains to the group that the child, David, is leaving the school soon and this will be the last time we will meet together with David in this setting. David is then asked to leave the room and return when someone calls for him. The group then get together to collect individual positive statements which describe something of David. Someone can have the task of writing everyone's statements down on paper. We often find the children will dress the paper up by putting things on like 'To David, it was good to have you in our group—good luck'. When all is complete someone calls David into the room to receive his positive suggestions. The group may or may not want David to guess who said what. That must be previously decided upon. David is allowed to take away his positive suggestions.

CONCLUSIONS

1. The positive suggestions are personal and apply to the one who is leaving, thus giving that child a feeling of well being.
2. The suggestions received give a measure of the impression which has been made on others.
3. Everyone acknowledges someone is leaving. If left alone this could be a difficult concept for children who have not yet made the 'grade'.
4. The paper with the suggestions remains with the leaver, so that the leaver takes a pleasing memory of the group.
5. By saying goodbye the leaver is making a statement to himself as well as the group. He is therefore preparing for the next step, the return to the family.

'Goodbye'

Everyone in the group sits in a circle and the leader explains that someone is leaving the group. Each child must then think of something to finish off the sentence, 'I would like to say goodbye to Janet and . . .' It must be emphasised that only positive statements must be made. In turn Janet can be given the opportunity to say goodbye to each child in the same way. If this is too much Janet could say a goodbye statement to the group as a whole.

CONCLUSION

These are much the same as for positive suggestion, but the leaving child also is given the opportunity to say a positive goodbye.

11   On being a member of the community

Most children of school age attend one or more extra-curricular activities during the week. This is invariably a group activity of some kind and may take the form of attending the Scouts or the Brownies or going to youth clubs or community centres. Attendance at these activities is optional, but children usually find themselves more than willing to attend as part of the general process of learning and socialisation. In areas of high unemployment or where there is a lack of social and recreational facilities, the youth clubs and community centres have come to represent a place where children can meet, and entertain themselves and be entertained while, at the same time, learning about themselves through each other and through the group experience.

The adults who work with children in these group activities are mainly volunteers and come from all walks of life and from different professions. The staff who run youth clubs and community centres may be social workers or youth workers. The premises in which these activities are based may be on local council property or in schools or church halls. The children usually do not have far to travel and perhaps the whole idea is that the activities are based centrally within the whole community and foster the idea of children belonging to that particular community. What follows, of course, is that the community mores then strongly apply, parents become involved and an atmosphere is created of belonging to a wider group in which there is a sense of accountability between the members.

The children who attend youth clubs and community centres come from different backgrounds and range from the highly socially able child to the slightly less well adjusted child. For some children attending the Brownies or the Scouts is only one aspect of an otherwise full life. For others their youth clubs or the community centres represent the only source of stimulation, learning and entertainment. These children may come from families in difficult circumstances, from single-parent families, or from families in which there is considerable material as well as emotional deprivation. For them the interaction with the peer group becomes as important as the interaction with the adults who are involved in these activities.

What then is the function of the group in the community. Clearly, as already mentioned in previous paragraphs, there is the educational benefits to be derived from such activities, as well as the entertainment value that the activities hold. Also, since these groups are based in the community, there is an emphasis on the concept of community living as well as encouraging the children to adopt the mores of the community. At a different level, these activities can be said to promote the psychological, social and emotional growth of the children and these aspects are highlighted in other chapters in the book. Another function of these group activities lies in the development of relationships between the adults and the children in these settings. Thus, whereas for some children this will have been a 'good' experience of relating to an adult, albeit an adult who occupies a peripheral position in the child's life, there will obviously be other children for whom this relationship occupies a central and important position in their lives.

The question that arises is to what extent should the adults who run these groups be consciously aware of the group function and to what extent should they consciously pursue these aims. The question that follows is whether the case may be made for all adult volunteers and paid workers alike to receive some kind of training in the running of these groups. There is no simple answer to these questions. At the same time it is clear that the majority of children are happy enough in themselves and with each other and do not require special attention. Equally, the majority of adult organisers of the activities will not wish to see their role as putting their charges under the microscope to examine their behaviour. That may well be regarded as a role for the professionals. There may be an argument for this kind of approach detracting from the spontaneity and fun in these activities and for it causing an uneven distribution of attention, with some children getting more attention from the adults than the others. There may be an anxiety that this kind of approach will arouse rivalries and bad feelings between the children that will in itself defeat the whole purpose of the exercise of putting the children together for an enjoyable time.

Perhaps the answer lies in the individual sensitivities and inclination of the adults concerned. Clearly there can be no compulsion to follow one or another approach so that all adults running groups could be expected to use sense, observation and empathy in dealing with children in their charge. Just one point may be made in this connection, as a reminder—if anyone needs reminding, that the group offers a tremendous opportunity to recognise the child in difficulty and where possible to offer that child help in the group context to cope with these difficulties.

We would now like to describe the highlights from one particular session of a community group activity that we observed and later to summarise our observation of this and other similar groups that we were very kindly allowed to sit in on, by the group leaders organising the activity.

THE CUBS

This is an all boys group ranging from eight to eleven years of age. There were five adults leading the group, three females and two males. In total the group lasted for one-and-a-half hours. It consisted of twenty boys including one boy who was mentally handicapped and he was well accepted by the group. Everyone, children and adults alike, all wore a uniform, so from early beginnings there was a feeling of conformity, leading to a sense of belonging.

On arrival the boys became engaged in unstructured play, and gradually the noise levels increased considerably alongside the energy output. However, it was not before one of the adults gave a special command to encourage the boys to sub-group into their sixes. At this point a structure was imposed and proceedings began. The cubs delivered a cub motto consisting of a salute and the hoisting of the flag. All members were seen to participate and it was all taken very seriously. These rituals added further to the feelings of identity and belonging to a group, and offered a structure which the group could easily relate to in a positive way.

After the motto a sense of anticipation built up around the groups, the noise levels increased and fidgeting started. However, the cubs were attentive and responded well when the adult suggested the next activity. A series of games followed, all very energetic, and for a bunch of lively boys it was obviously meeting their needs.

The boys were encouraged to work within the boundaries of the game and any deviations from this resulted in being gently but firmly redirected by the adults. The ordinary, everyday football featured largely in most of the games that were offered and the boys seemed to identify readily with this symbol of the national game! The last of the games was a competition with prizes for correct answers. This game encouraged a more cognitive thought by working out anagrams of football teams, it also encouraged co-operativeness because the boys had to work in their sub-groups and consequently the focus was on the team rather than on the individual. Therefore, there was less chance of individuals feeling alone and inadequate within the competition.

On the whole the children made their own sub-groups by working in twos and threes. There was also a lot of interaction between child and adult leader. The sixes themselves were all given common things to do throughout the evening, but as previously said the boys preferred to work in smaller groups.

Over the weeks of attending cubs, certain tasks have to be achieved such as badges which may include working on these at home or school, therefore creating further interactions and interests outwith the main stem of the cub group. The boys also have an opportunity to attend a camp. This leads onto involvement of daily living tasks and responsibility towards their fellow cubs.

At the end of the group a cub scout prayer was said which indicated it was time for home. At this point the boys seemed relaxed and left the building in groups which was a contrast to their arrival when they arrived alone.

OBSERVATION OF OTHER GROUPS

In most groups, starting was an important eventful issue. It was at this point that a structure emerged which gave rise to the children having some identity with the group and a safe environment to spend the next one-and-a-half to two hours. Most groups offered a 'warm up' exercise. Children arrive at a group with a whole range of feelings, anxieties, and different energy levels and a 'warm up' exercise in terms of a common group game, can help to reduce any anxiety, allowing a feeling of well-being to develop within the group. This will also serve to help the children participate more appropriately in further activities. One 'warm up' game observed was called 'Ladders'. Each child had to find a partner and the partners were given a number. The children sat facing their partners with their feet touching. This essentially formed a ladder made up of legs. When the leader shouted out a number the partner whom the number belonged to had to negotiate the ladder by jumping in the space between the legs and then return to their place, each trying to get back before the other. From this 'warm up' game the sheer physical effort of the game reduces the energy levels and will ultimately reduce any anxiety which may have been present. From observation it was noted that there were different levels of participation and different levels of dexterity. However, because the game was the focus it allowed full participation, encouraging interaction and therefore building up a feeling of cohesion and belonging with all the children.

ON BEING A MEMBER OF THE COMMUNITY 115

Often children like to have a familiar structure to give them some stability and allow them to feel relaxed enough to deal with the next event. Certainly this was the case, with the Cubs and Brownies. When the 'warm up' game had finished the children assembled and became involved with their various rituals. It was at this point the children settled and became quietly co-operative. The adults had full charge of their children, giving rise to a feeling of security with the adults rather than a fear of authority. Amongst these rituals the children at various levels had their own parts to play which resulted in giving a certain amount of responsibility to the child and allowing a modelling process to develop for the younger or newer members of the group.

From the sub-grouping which emerged when, for instance, the Brownies had to get into their sixes, it was evident that a sense of recognition and identity to their group had developed, adding an element of competition with the other groups. This was fostered by the leader who looked for the best turned out sixes or the quietest sixes. While competitiveness itself can be quite anxiety provoking, in these groups the competitiveness had a positive focus and was healthy in terms of the group sharing and the trying out of their own interactional skills.

A great deal of variety was included in these various groups from everyone involved in group games, to small group games, to task orientated groups, to individuals working independently on various badges. The inclusion of tasks for the groups offered a chance to learn new practical, creative skills and produce an end product which could be proudly shared with others, thus offering a boost to a child's self-esteem. For individuals working on badges the opportunity was given to try out new ideas or build upon previously learnt skills which often offered a new challenge. On completion of the badge or task, a sense of achievement and feeling of satisfaction was evident. It was also something tangible and could be taken home to show the family. It was usual for more than one child to work on a badge thereby allowing further development of positive peer group relations and sharing, because the focus of the activity had a common theme.

Many of the group games we observed were quite energetic which seemed to fit in with the mood and the needs of the group. The opportunity to verbally express themselves in a game counteracted the periods when the leader needed moments of silence. When watching a group of boys between the age of six to seven years playing their games, one could detect their feelings from their expressions. Their expressions portrayed a mixture of anxious participation and involvement to having fun and looking happy. It was whilst watching these boys that we noted the usefulness of peer group pressure. One child who was finding it difficult to join in had his peer group shout at him to hurry and he began to conform. By the use of peer group pressure the control stays within the group rather than putting the leader in an authoritarian role. Seeing the effectiveness of peer group pressure, we were also very aware of the effectiveness of the children relating to their group leaders. As stated previously, the leader was not just a figure of authority, but someone who could be relied upon for individual needs as well as for group needs. The children had permission to relate to their leaders in a relaxed manner; to use their leaders to sort out their problems; to look for sympathy if they felt hurt; to look for praise for something they had achieved; to step in when authority was needed and make the situation feel secure again; above all to know that whatever happened they would not be rejected.

All groups come to an end and the ending is as important as the beginning. After experiencing energy and enthusiasim, children need a quite time to allow these feelings to subside, whereupon the children will leave the group in a relaxed and positive manner. This was achieved largely by imposing a structure on the children and expecting them to conform to a particular theme. The theme varied from saying a prayer together or engaging in a very quiet exercise which was common to the group ending.

12 Groups for the sexually abused child

ROSEMARIE MUSGRAVE

Sexual abuse of children has been forced onto everybody's awareness in recent years and has alarmed all involved professions. The need to respond positively to allegations has developed guidelines about close and productive co-operation between the professions. Workers in all fields are receiving training to help them deal with these complex and anxiety provoking allegations. People often have to learn very fast. The pressures on all workers are often extreme both in terms of time and complexities of the issues that have to be dealt with in an increasingly public arena. Decisions have to be made; the abuse has to be stopped; the child needs to be protected. Once the decisions about the allegations have been made, the pressure changes or eases considerably. Often case conferences suggest that work should be done with the child, but this is usually left to the individual workers. Experience has shown that the pressure on all workers to investigate and assess has now been matched by pressure to treat the needs of children and their caretakers. The word therapy and treatment are used but little is available to the victims. We all seem to know so little about what helps children. We become particularly concerned about the needs of the younger children. Workers are less sure of their roles with them, when the use of language for the 'talking it through' type of therapy does not appear appropriate.

We found how little is known in this country about treatment of the young child, and could not find any research that evaluates the impact of treatment on children of different ages and developmental stages or of different modalities of treatment. Most books consider a family systems approach as preferred method of treatment, usually by multi-disciplinary teams meeting with various sub-groups of family members. Besides this family orientated approach, group therapy has been advocated for adolescent victims of sexual abuse, but Kee MacFarlane *et al.* describe work with younger children. I have attempted to help children who had been separated from their families of origin on an individual basis when they presented problems following sexual abuse, mainly working on play therapy lines. As referral for treatment of young children increased, we decided to explore group work as a chosen model. The purpose of the group would be to help the children with their experiences, make them feel less isolated, guilty and responsible for the abuse and, hopefully, give them greater confidence in general, but particularly regarding further abusive situations.

THE TREATMENT ISSUES

There is still considerable debate about whether all child sex abuse victims will suffer from all the issues listed below. The severity of abuse obviously varies greatly too. Only future rigorous research will give up adequate certainty. In the meantime, in any therapeutic relationship we need to give all the issues listed below equal importance and, therefore, the order of the list is quite arbitrary. S. Sgroi has a similar list:

1. Impaired ability to trust/inappropriate trust.
2. Confusion over sexuality and affection.
3. Self protection.
4. The 'damaged goods' syndrome and low self-esteem and poor social skills/attention-seeking behaviour.
5. Disclosure.
6. Repressed anger and hostility.
7. Guilt/sense of responsibility for what happened.
8. Fear.
9. Blurred role boundaries and role confusion.
10. Depression.

These are the main issues. We had to face our own feelings of outrage about the children's trauma and face the difficulty of breaking the general taboo about talking to young children about sexual matters. We worried about the balance we needed to strike between openness and incitement to even more sexualised behaviour. We seriously considered our necessary contact both with the children's social workers and particularly the caretakers. Before and after the last session of each group, we invited the caretakers to talk to us. These meetings gave us evidence of how much the relationship of natural mother to their daughter becomes distorted following the disclosure of sexual abuse. We have regretted the fact that simultaneous groups for the caretakers were not possible. In future, we would try even harder to offer this service.

Our first group was largely based on the Great Ormond Street model. This is a six-week, well prepared programme of weekly sessions where the children are taught self-protection via assertiveness training, some sex education and re-education about good, bad and 'icky' touching, and helped to tell adults about dangerous experiences. The whole programme is very much a teaching programme with excellent flash-cards and good instructions to the workers. In our pre-group planning, we each week made our own programme and then checked it out with the Great Ormond Street model. This process gave us a sense of independence, but also great confidence that we were on the 'right' lines. It was good to be able to be confirmed in this way.

The six girls referred to the group had been sexually abused, or were suspected of having been sexually abused by either the father, or mother's cohabitee. They were mainly referred because their behaviour had given rise to some quite serious concern, rather than because they were sexually abused. Two of the girls had themselves abused other children, one quite seriously. Our criterion was mainly one of age, we wanted them to be between six and eight, and ended up with two five-year-olds, two six-year-olds, one eight-year-old and one ten-year-old.

The groups were run by the same team of two female and one male worker, all social workers but working normally in different settings. It is clearly necessary to feel comfortable with one's co-workers in this area of work. During the long planning stage, the female co-worker, Fiona, and I got to know each other very well; it was harder for the male worker, Andy, to join us at a later stage. We wanted to present a healthy male-female model to the children, so we particularly valued our male colleague to give us this balance. In our second mixed gender group, we valued his presence even more. As the needs of sexually abused children are acute, we hoped three workers would offer more time to listen to them, but also would cope better in case of the absence of one of the workers.

Already after two sessions of the first group, we began to become uncertain of our chosen approach, and geared ourselves towards the next group, that would last for ten weeks and, hopefully, be quite different. We felt the routine of the programme forced the pace far too much and gave us all the control over pace, material and content. As we became more relaxed ourselves, we could be more sensitive to the children's pace, listen much better and vary the response to their needs. The same workers managed to stick with this second group, so our learning developed on a team basis.

For group two, we had referrals for three girls and one boy, two of the girls had also experienced group one. We could find no reason to exclude Tom aged five. The girls were eight, six and five. We quite seriously considered the gender issue of group members. The developmental stage of the children needs to be assessed with great care. We felt strongly that single sex groups are much more appropriate for adolescent victims, or even pre-adolescents, but with young children we feel the groups can be mixed, but obviously this depends in part on the composition of the group. The gender issue was discussed each time Tom misbehaved! We are not sure that we have the answer. We hoped Tom would manage as the only boy. Our experience showed that the girls and Tom accepted each other and Tom clearly benefited from the group experience.

As with all group work, much of our time was taken up with the pre-planning, both in advance of the groups but particularly before each session. As none of us are teachers, the control element needed good preparation. We had the use of a large room with some play material, like a Wendy House, a sand-tray and Doll's House, tables and chairs, bean-bags, blackboard, overhead-video cameras, but also hand-held video camera and monitor; art material, dressing-up clothes and glove puppets were materials we felt we needed. Children learn through play, you cannot just talk with them. We needed to create a balance between fun and learning. We made up a collection of trust games, particularly suited to younger children and preferably with lots of body contact, movement and noise. At the end of each session, once the work part was done, we always had biscuits and orange-juice before free play.

The children of the groups that we have run have helped us enormously to understand the issues related to child sex abuse, deprivation and hurt and we want to express our gratitude and ensure total anonymity by changing all the names and important historical details.

I now want to explore some of the treatment issues listed before with material from our group experience.

TRUST

Generally all groups should be designed to engender trust. The place and time should be absolutely secure from any changes and should feel private and safe. We had toilets close by, so the children did not have to cross the path of others. Transport was organised by the children's social workers. The welcome and the sense of importance each member receives must be considered. When one of the children could not attend we sent them a card to make sure they felt they were missed. We planned our behaviour around respect for them and accepted their choices as much as we could.

We started each group with learning all our names through playing a 'name game' with a ball. We created a group poster. We took polaroid pictures of the children and stuck these on the poster where they wanted them. The group poster was there each week. We hoped this would give them a sense that the room belonged to them. We decided the group had to have rules for the sessions. No hurting each other or us, no breaking of property, no leaving before the end of the session. We explained confidentiality and our wish to keep their stories safe. We explained the video cameras as being something we needed as a means of helping them. In the first session, we gave them the reason for the meetings and told them for how long we would meet and that we would have an outing on the last session that they could choose. The reason for meeting we repeated in the second session as we felt they might have been too bewildered by so many new things. We said, 'Each of you has had something nasty, unpleasant or rude happen to you and we want to try and help you feel better about this.'

Repeated routines develop trust, like the 'news' at the beginning of each session when the adults participate as equals and when we each talked only when the duck had been passed to us. This was also our attempt to calm down the excited babble. We also wished to establish trust in the group leaders, so that each person could be sure of having their turn at whatever was going on. Sitting down on the floor or bean-bags also made us more equal and gave us some security in a new and uncertain world.

We always planned the content of the sessions, at first with quite fixed programmes. This gave us confidence as none of us had run groups for sexually abused children before. I had had some experience of groups with adolescents. For the second group we also planned the sessions, but in a less structured way. This gave us time for individual work within the group context.

In general we were amazed how quickly the children seemed to trust us, and then we had to learn how superficial and inappropriate this trust sometimes was. In an early session we asked them to draw their family. They found this very hard. One little girl would only draw herself and mummy, another only her foster-family. On reflection, I felt they could not trust us yet with their real families with all the attendant hurts and confusions. Later when more trust was established, we heard of the daddies in prison. In a later group, we managed the same task much better. Quite different trust had been established and after a puppet play the children were asked to draw what they liked. They produced vivid pictures of freely expressed feelings about imaginary characters. One six-year-old girl drew a king's castle that nearly covered all the paper, at the narrow edge a girl stood outside this high castle wall with a very sad mouth. An eight-year-old drew a cat and the horrible dog the cat was frightened of. Each child had his/her work kept in a folder and at the end of all the sessions they took this home.

The inappropriate trust was shown when one five-year-old girl attempted far too close contact with Andy. We explored her behaviour with her and showed her how risky it was.

The trust games were often great romps. We used them as ice-breakers but also to talk of the feelings they raised in the children.

We wanted to help the children learn to trust their own feelings and give them frequent opportunities to make choices. We would then look with them at the outcome of their choice and how this affected them and others and, if necessary, learn from the feedback of the other children. Grabbing all the biscuits might be such an opportunity. In the first group we used the hand-held video and quick replay on the monitor to show them how they could make their expressions more congruent with their statements: they needed to practice many times how to tell somebody to leave them alone and to test their new-found assertiveness. They loved seeing themselves on TV.

CONFUSION OVER SEXUALITY AND AFFECTION

The sexually abused children need honest and straightforward help with their boundaries that have been thoroughly confused. Adults had told the children that sexual touching was all right, but then told them to keep this secret. Their own senses had been involved in ways that had excited, but also had hurt them. They had wanted the affection but not the sexual touching.

In this area of work the anatomically correct dolls were a great help. The children recognised them as similar to the ones used in the investigation process. They knew that the dolls needed undressing before their uniqueness became apparent. These dolls are large rag-dolls with nice velcro-fastening clothes that are easy to undress. They come in sets of two adults and two children, one of each sex. The adult dolls have pubic and under-arm hair, breasts, penis and scrotum. Anuses and vaginas look like continuous seams, but on probing become a slit that is silk lined and able to accommodate a finger or penis. All the dolls have round silk-lined mouths. Most of the children were giggly as they undressed the dolls. They were embarrassed by our presence and our willingness to be open. We asked for names of body parts and they needed help to include the ordinary ones like noses and toes!

When we made a poster of all the names they could think of for private parts, we found they gradually relaxed and the embarrassed giggling stopped. They seemed pleased to add to the list, fairy, willie, down there, boobs. We told them how each family has often their own names, and how some words become rude swear words. We also helped them to the professional words like vagina and penis. In each group we found all the children became quite open in talking about these private words, and we respected whatever they offered. One girl called out 'flowerpot' and touched herself between her legs, making the meaning very obvious. After the sharing of words, the children looked relieved and we all dressed the dolls again. We talked often with them about what they thought was private and what part of the body somebody else could touch, then enlarged this to the types of touching: good, bad and 'icky', and went over the same ground again and again. Some children had real problems over the idea of who owns their body. We explored the issue of ownership in a general context and then asked them who owned their body. Elsa, aged five, got quite upset that we did not really agree that Mummy owned her body. 'But I want her to', she shouted. So we had to explain this gently to her. As three of the five-year-olds had already become abusers themselves, we had to develop the touch issue further, so that they understood they could not touch other people without their consent. All the children were intensely keen on physical affection. We tried to channel this need into games that included permitted touching, rather than respond to their need. We always talked about what seemed to be going on and explored with them the possible risks involved. We continued to be concerned about some of the children whose hunger for affection may again expose them to further abuse.

SELF PROTECTION

We tried to tackle this issue from all sorts of angles. Only time will tell how successful we have been.

The 'No game' was fun and noisy. All of us formed a circle and then crouched down, humming only. As we slowly rose, the 'no' became louder until we stood up fully, with determined faces and arms outstretched yelling 'NO'. This we repeated in several sessions, but we became aware that not all the children liked the noise.

We talked a lot about risky situations and asked them what they could do, and developed this into role plays with the hand-held video camera and the monitor. We asked the children to help the acting person if things became difficult. Teachers seem to be universally preferred as confidants and the children all thought they could find a teacher to tell. Some had clearly been told to go up to a policeman and disclose their secret this way but they had given no real thought to how they could make a contact. We then gave them many chances to persist with an uninterested or disbelieving adult. They had to learn to become quite assertive with the 'Mums' or teachers, shouting in the end: 'Please listen'. In the safety of the group setting and feeling very confident, some of the children had quite unrealistic ideas about tackling the perpetrator. They were reminded of the size difference and their possible danger.

On reflection, we found it very interesting that in our first group we focused on the sex abuse coming much more from outside the family, so the exercises included self protection in relation to the man in the road or park or the baby-sitter, in spite of us knowing that the children had experienced the abuse much more from parent figures. We began to realise how hard we ourselves found it to discuss the inter-familial abuse. We felt we needed to overcome this reluctance to be able to seriously attempt to help the children. Maybe the puppets helped as much as the children.

LOW SELF-ESTEEM AND POOR SOCIAL SKILLS

We saw many examples of these issues. Sheila, aged eight, always looked very uncared for. Her skin and clothes were dirty. We knew her to have been severely abused. She grasped for everything, interrupted and was quick to quarrel and demand attention. She had come to our first group and we were very uncertain how much she had gained. Then we heared that she had been further abused by her mother's new cohabitee and was re-referred to our second group. When Andy, the co-worker, welcomed her saying something nice to her, she replied, 'No, I don't look nice, I am ugly'. The coldness of this statement was hard to take. She said it with firm conviction and a straight serious face and when Andy tried to reassure her, she indicated by her expression that nothing would move her from her opinion.

In session two, Sheila had listened with interest to the second instalment of the puppet play of a cat disclosing gradually to an accepting teacher Miss Owl. She then drew a cat and kept on saying, 'This cat feels dirty, she keeps on washing herself but she cannot get clean'. In a later session, when the children were dressing up with a great variety of fancy colourful clothes, she was very unwilling to join in. We gently offered her different garments and hats. With resignation she eventually took the clown's hat and put this on. While the others were having fun, we talked with her about how sad she looked and she said she did not feel pretty. We talked about this too. Very gradually she relaxed a little and by the end of the session, still wearing the clown's hat, she joined with the others and had some fun. We took photos of them all for their folders. The group members became very important in confirming each child. Sheila progressed well through the weeks.

In session eight, we had prepared many labels of coloured gummed paper, each with a positive word on it. Each child was asked to make their own poster by writing their name boldly on gummed paper and sticking this on. We then asked them to suggest good characteristics for each other: kind, generous, great, pretty, good listener, caring . . . Then each child had to stick the chosen word on their paper. Sheila amazed us. She made up a figure with all the labels around the centre of her name. She told us it was a girl and the girl felt good. We talked about the attributes that she so confidently stuck on to her poster. She clearly had achieved some change in her image of herself.

Tom, aged five, found it sometimes very hard to contribute. We then wondered how much his being the only boy was a serious problem for him. He told us in his news many unlikely boastful stories and we tried to talk with him about how much he wanted to be such a tough and nasty boy. He was another child that did not feel good about himself. He painted an enormous muddy mess and added more colours to the large circular figure. We talked with him about this dark and frightening feeling which he was trying to convey to us. Later we heard from his mother that he had for a long time been a very quiet, shy boy, particularly reticent about undressing and getting into the bath. She is an experienced mother and was very unhappy about this. After the end of the groups, she told us that gradually during the time we met with him he changed, became out-going, cheeky and has now no problems about undressing.

Molly's feeling bad took on very physical symptoms. Early on she had been car-sick by the time she arrived with us. Gradually she developed a sick person's role in the group. She managed to make herself sick one week after a drink of water, but in spite of this never refused biscuits and orange. We gave her and all the children as much attention as we could, always talked about what they and we were doing. Molly needed loads of attention. She even managed to worry her Mum who discussed her withdrawal from the group as an option. When we supported Mum and suggested that at best she should ignore the tall stories, and again invited Molly, she came without too much talk of sickness and a great deal of hunger for all the goodies. Molly gradually had to learn to listen to the other children and give them her proper attention too.

We talked at different times about how they wanted to be different, how they could get an adult's attention and how to protect themselves. We helped them to accept compliments from each other and try and find something good to say to each other. It is very hard to say how far the children's low self-esteem and their poor social skills were attributable to the sexual abuse they had experienced and how far to some very poor parenting.

DISCLOSURE

In our first group, disclosure had been a difficult grey area. Some of the children said something when the babble was at its loudest and would then be reluctant to repeat it, and we did not push. We were left very uncertain. We felt some wanted to speak and were not sure of the trust, but we were also concerned about the effect any horrendous details might have on children whose abuse had only been alleged but not proven, or who had experienced a less severe form of abuse.

In the second group and after much thought, we decided to deal with disclosure issue through glove-puppet plays ourselves. We would never ask for, but give great attention to any of the children's disclosures. This plan worked very well indeed. 'Suzi the cat' acted out her reluctance to speak to teacher 'Miss Owl' and in several little episodes we could explore whatever issues we felt uppermost in the group.

After the first session, we heard from Tom's social worker how good it was to hear that he had disclosed the abuse which up to then had only been suspected abuse. He had told both his mother at length and also the social worker. Separately, he said to each, 'Do you want to know my secret?', and had then given them all the details. In the group he was a very intent listener to the puppet role plays, although at first appeared to be disinterested. When in week two, we asked the children about the role play, he could repeat word for word what had been said by both Suzi and Miss Owl.

In session five, we asked the children if they would like to be Suzi, the cat. The workers had decided there would, in turn, be a teacher Miss Owl and a Mr Owl. Three of the children were definitely keen to take part. They all had long stories.

Molly cat told Miss Owl about how she was frightened of Richard who visits her mother. This just poured out of her, hardly needing the imaginary cat role. She talked of violence and sexual abuse and she seemed to talk of both herself and her mother being victims. She became quite intense as the story emerged, speaking very quickly and seemingly recalling separate incidents. The whole picture of the nature of the abuse was quite hard to follow. Miss Owl tried to clarify and asked Molly to become more specific.

Then Mr Owl asked Sheila cat if she was all right and why she was not going out with the rest of the children. Sheila said she felt sad. Mr Owl suggested she go to play to cheer herself up, but she said she did not feel like it. At this point Mr Owl asked her what was wrong. By this time Sheila's voice was very serious and sad. She said she was frightened because Mum's boyfriend had been touching her. Mr Owl said, 'What do you mean by frightened?' Sheila said that he touches the top of her legs and her privates. Mr Owl said, 'This is very sad, we must try and do something about this', but without prompting she, in a trembling voice, then disclosed a whole string of sexual touching and activities.

Mr Owl by then asked Sheila cat if she wanted to come closer, and then he asked her how she felt about this man. She said she hated him and Mr Owl asked her if she could say all this to the police. Mr Owl found it difficult to know how to finish this experience as Sheila had shared so much.

It again became evident how much we need the close support of co-workers. Fiona could say to the group how well Sheila cat had done to tell things that we all find difficult and sad to talk about. Sheila's story affected the whole group, workers and children. Mr Owl found maintaining his role difficult because of the extent of the disclosure. This Sheila cat story helped both Tom and Lena to tell their stories. All the children were praised about how hard they had worked. We wondered how the children had coped, they certainly had deserved their drinks and biscuits. The workers felt that it had taken the development of trust in the previous four weeks to enable the children to be so open and honest. The workers later checked that the children's social workers were already aware of all the allegations.

REPRESSED ANGER AND HOSTILITY

Tom was quite angry in one session, he eventually had to be separated by Andy from the rest of the group and calmed down. He vividly painted large bold messes and to help him express some of these feelings we gave him boxing-gloves and held up a bean-bag for him to punch. We suggested he gave voice to his feelings but did not push him to express names or any other disclosing statements. It was interesting that he always gave it to 'him' with real power.

Sheila expressed her anger with paint. She took a long time to paint a figure with great care, finally adding an appendage between the trouser legs. She explained that this was his 'privates' and that 'he will get it in there'. She she finished the rest of the figure she used her brush like an attacking instrument and with short hard stabs she added red paint to the penis, then began to flick the red paint all over the large picture. She became quite engrossed in this and was very reluctant to stop. In fact, she continued while eating biscuits and drinking her orange. We helped her to voice her feelings and she enjoyed expressing her anger and fury. There was never any doubt about who she was attacking.

Molly talked of knives under pillows for protection and about a man friend of her mother's. It never became quite clear where fantasy ended and reality began.

Lena talked with anger and hostility about big boys.

GUILT/SENSE OF RESPONSIBILITY FOR WHAT HAPPENED

The experiences of adult and adolescent victims indicate that the sense of guilt and responsibility for the abuse is carried by the victim in a very persistent way and usually against all logic. We expected to have to give these issues a lot of attention.

In our groups we were surprised by how these young children did not seem to carry this guilt. We frequently heard them say that it was the fault of the man, and then they would express open anger. We think that this was the result of their own social workers' help, particularly as the children had to wait for up to eighteen months before the first group became available. We are also wondering if this sense of guilt develops over time as the children become more aware of the moral implications. The abuse was always accompanied by demands to keep silent about it and the children were threatened if they disclosed. Tom was told by his Dad that he would kill him if he told about it, and the children certainly experienced fear of consequences, fear of breaking these rules, of not doing as they were told.

We felt we still wanted them to experience in a very factual way the power and size differential between themselves and a man. To make this very apparent we created a life-sized cut out figure of a man and stood the children against this. We also told them that they were right not to resist as this would have been dangerous as they themselves were so much smaller than the grown-up. When we talked about the responsibility for what had happened to them, they thought we were silly and used the cut out figure like a growth chart to show their size, and again expressed open anger towards the perpetrators.

GROUPS FOR THE SEXUALLY ABUSED CHILD

We are aware that these children will at a later stage again need reassurance and confirmation that sexual abuse is always the responsibility of the perpetrator.

In the space available, I have covered only some of the treatment issues, our work in the groups touched on all of them.

Endings are very important. Many sessions we ended with each in turn saying what we had disliked and later in turn what we had liked in this session. Other sessions we ended with each person saying something complimentary about the person next to us. We needed to help the children accept compliments.

Although we had prepared them for the fact that these sessions would come to an end, some found this hard to accept. The last session became the promised outing. They were fully involved in choosing and planning the outing. They found this difficult, but a food source was each time top of the list. The last group we took to a large park with several play areas and an adventure play-ground. We were equipped with sixteen crisp packets and they were all gradually eaten. Although they were very hungry, some shared with the Canada geese and ducks. On the play equipment, boastful Tom revealed to us how timid he still is. With much help, he gradually gained trust and confidence in himself during the afternoon. The children became very possessive about the attention of the workers. We had to be scrupulously fair with our listening and watching. Even singing at times became difficult as the children could not agree who was the leader. We talked about this with them and they could then chose a way out of the dilemma.

The group ended up with dirty hands and knees in MacDonald's and consumed an extraordinary quantity and mixture of food and drink, some as if they had not been fed for weeks.

As we dropped them off ourselves, we gave them each in turn their folders, with all their work, the lovely photos we took of them and a few little gifts, the reality dawned on them that this was the end of our time together. We again confirmed how hard they had worked over the many weeks, how much they had learnt and how we hoped they would cope much better in any future risky situation. We told them what great kids they were and how much we wished them all the best.

Appendix I

SOME GAMES TO PLAY WITH THE CHILDREN 5–10

The Name of the Game:
Purpose: To introduce and memorise names.
Method: Sit in a circle, pass ball and each person receiving the ball says their name very clearly. Then the ball is thrown to any person and the receiver must say the thrower's name.

Group yell: No:
Purpose: To release tension, to warm up, trust building.
Method: Group huddle together in crouching position. Leader begins low hum. As the group begins to rise slowly, 'No' is said with the sound level also rising, ending with everyone standing up with determined faces, arms outstretched yelling 'no'.

Pile up:
Purpose: Legitimate body contact leading to discussion.
Method: Group members lie on their stomachs and close their eyes. All start crawling towards central point and they meet. They crawl over each other until a pile starts to form in the centre. When the pile is complete they all open their eyes. Teacher helps them to express what they felt in their position.

Toesies
Purpose: Touching and co-operative play, trust.
Method: Children take off their shoes. Partners simply lie stretched out on the floor, feet to feet or big toe to big toe, and attempt to roll across the floor keeping their toes touching throughout.

Beachball or Balloon Balance
Purpose: Closeness, co-operative play, trust.
Method: One ball or balloon to two children. Without using hands they can find out how many ways there are to balance the

ball between them. (Head to head, side to side, stomach, back.)

While they attempt to move around holding the ball in different ways they can be asked to do other things with their hands, like touch knees, toes, both squat. Obstacles to negotiate can be a further lesson, or balancing the ball between four people.

The Scribble in the air and then on paper

Purpose: Relaxing, loosening, freeing.

Method: Ask the children to stand apart, close their eyes and then to stretch their arms as high, wide and low as they can, and imagine themselves to be drawing a high scribble picture in front of them on imaginary paper and with imaginary crayons in each hand. Every part and all corners are to be filled.

Then sitting down ask them to repeat this on a piece of paper, and then ask them to find forms in their scribble that suggest a picture and ask them to outline these. Then talk about what they have found.

Appendix II

Puppet Play of Disclosure   First of several scenes

Equipment: Two glove puppets, a cushion or bean-bag as scenery. (We had a cat and an owl.)

Suzi: 'I am Suzi and I am very unhappy.'
Children: 'Who is that?'
Suzi: 'I am Suzi, the cat, and I am very unhappy. Something bad has happened to me and I don't know what to do about it.'
Children: 'Can we have a turn?'
Suzi: *(ignoring the interruption):* 'I really don't know to whom I can talk about it. I think when I go to school I will talk to my teacher.'
Suzi: *(introducing the Owl):* 'This is my teacher.'
Children: *(Laughing).*
Suzi: 'My teacher is Miss Owl. I don't really know how to talk to Miss Owl with all the other kids. I think I'll wait until they are all outside in the playground.'
Suzi: 'Miss Owl, can I have a talk with you please?'
Miss Owl: 'What do you want to talk about, Suzi?'
Suzi: 'I find it really difficult, Miss Owl. I have been thinking about talking with you for a long time, but I don't know how to start.'
Miss Owl: 'Well, why don't we sit down somewhere comfortable and then you can try and tell me something.'
(Both sitting on the bean-bag)
Miss Owl: 'This is really quite comfortable, Suzi, shall we sit down side by side?' *(facing the children)*
Miss Owl: 'What do you want to talk to me about?'
Suzi: 'Well, Miss Owl, I really feel quite shy about what I want to say. You see, it is something to do with my Daddy.'
Miss Owl: 'What is the matter with your Daddy?'
Suzi: 'Well . . . Nothing is the matter with my Daddy, but you see sometimes when everybody else is out of the house he wants me to sit very close to him and I get a funny feeling.'
Miss Owl: 'What sort of a funny feeling?'
Suzi: 'Well . . . I don't know, somewhere inside me . . . a funny sort of icky feeling.'

Miss Owl: 'Where do you get that feeling?'
Suzi: 'Well . . . kind of all over, sort of, right deep down inside me.'
Miss Owl: 'What does your Daddy do when you get that icky feeling?'
Suzi: 'He sort of tries to touch me.'
Miss Owl: 'I am really glad you told me, Suzi. I think we need to do something about it.'
One of the children: 'The cat did not look sad.'
R.M.: 'I think her voice was sad. What do you think . . .?'

Some addresses for further information

Eileen Uizard: Department of Psychological Medicine, Great Ormond Street, London
Self Esteem and Personal Safety, a guide for professionals working with sexually abused children.

Anatomically Correct Dolls:
Show and Tell Dolls, 23 Marley Coombe Road, Camelsdale, Hazlemere, Surrey, GU27 3SN (Tel. 0428 4402)

Books
Kee MacFarlane *et al.*, *Sexual Abuse of Young Children* (Holt, Rinehart & Winston, 1986)
Jean Goodwin, *Sexual Abuse—Incest Victims and their Families* (Wright, Bristol 1982)
David Pitters, *We Can Say No* (Beaver Books, 1986)
Michelle Morris, *If I should die before I wake* (Souvenir Press, 1983)
Violet Oaklander, *Windows to our Children* (Real People Press, 1978)
Donna Brandes and Howard Phillips, *Gamester's Handbook* (Hutchinson, 1978)
Terry Orlick, *Co-operative Sports and Games Book* (Writers and Readers Publishing Co-operative, 1982)